Praise for HOPE BEYOND FIBROIDS

"HOPE BEYOND FIBROIDS: Stories of Miracle Babies & the Journey to Motherhood will help women everywhere lead fierce, faith-defining lives with the kind of immeasurable tenacity that silences all fears!"

—Mikki Taylor | Author, Speaker, Creative Strategist

"There are times when life is testing you, your patience, and ultimately your faith—times when you can feel as if you are alone in your struggles. Even when you are a person of faith, you can feel as if God is testing you and you alone. HOPE BEYOND FIBROIDS reminds you that no matter what you are going through, you are blessed, you can handle it, and there are rich lessons in your pain. This book celebrates not just the miracle of life but the affirmations of faith."

—Lisa Price | Founder, Carol's Daughter

"I found myself choking back tears and whispering, 'Amen!' with each story told in HOPE BEYOND FIBROIDS: Stories of Miracle Babies & the Journey to Motherhood. This is an amazingly inspirational telling of real women's journeys rooted in honesty, transparency, and raw emotion. Sometimes the difficulties encountered are too much to digest, then miraculously the joy of the journey shines through. I fervently believe that we overcome by the blood of the Lamb and the words of our testimony. This book is a cool drink in the heat of the battle; and the much needed encouragement for every woman who is fighting to be a mother."

Turner Bell | Host, ARISE News,
Veterinarian

D1157654

"*Gessie is the hero we needed to bring the fibroid conversation cen-ter stage. She encouraged me, and if you read this you too will find hope on these pages. Whether you are a mother or not, praying for a child, or beyond childbearing, just having access to* **HOPE BEYOND FIBROIDS** *is the invitation we needed to have the conversation about a painful, embarrassing, and emotional journey. All women should read this book and share it with at least one other sister friend!*"

—Dee Marshall | Founder, Girlfriends Pray Ministries

"*Kudos to Gessie Thompson as she shares her story—and those of fifteen other inspiring women—in* **HOPE BEYOND FIBROIDS**. *As a woman who has successfully overcome infertility issues, I commend her for bringing forth a miracle baby while facing her mountainous obstacles and fears with faith and determination. I pray other women will read this book and be encouraged as they walk through their chal-lenges and experiences. Sometimes we must push through the problem and learn the lessons so we can fully experience God's Grace on the other side.*"

—Debra Peek-Haynes
Author of The Beginner's Guide to Healthy Living
First Lady, Friendship West Baptist Church

"**HOPE BEYOND FIBROIDS** *is a message that I am person-ally passionate about. My mother suffered severely from fibroids and would always pray over my womb when I became pregnant with my children. The stories in this book remind me of a mother's prayer. Gessie*

Thompson shares her powerful message that miracles do happen if we pray and stand in faith. I highly recommend this book for the women who are suffering silently. This book will heal your heart and speak to your soul."

—Lucinda Cross | Celebrity Life Coach
Bestselling Author, *The Art of Activation*

"Are you ready for something captivating? **HOPE BEYOND FIBROIDS** offers accounts of sixteen women fighting fibroids, infertility, and seemingly impossible complications to receive their miracle babies. Gessie Thompson has written a book that's informative and accessible, as it combines inspiring stories of HOPE and INSPIRATION. I am in awe of her determination, strength, faith, and spirit as she persevered through the trials and kept believing—thus beating the odds in becoming a mommy! Thompson's real-life narrative is sure to empower, educate, and inspire all women."

—Angelia L. White | Publisher & CEO
Hope for Women magazine

"Our capacity to be a beacon of light for others in the world is often activated AFTER overcoming our own seasons of personal darkness. My friend Gessie Thompson COURAGEOUSLY and transparently shares her 'journey of hope' in **HOPE BEYOND FIBROIDS** so that other women may be inspired to get through another day, another moment, another breath on their own path to motherhood! The fact

that Gessie chose to share not only her story but those of others is indic-
ative of her loving spirit and understanding that while we can go
through difficult days alone, it is so much more bearable when we do
it together!"

—Dr. Vikki Johnson | Chaplain, Speaker,
Author & Media Executive

"Although this book is written to encourage women who have to walk
a difficult fertility journey, after reading it, I realize it is for EVERY
person faced with any challenge on this journey we call life. Trav-
eling through Gessie's quest to get to her miracle Nia, I rejoiced in
her highs and I couldn't find my breath during her lows. Reading
through the many stories of hope, I was encouraged by their unshake-
able faith, strengthened by their tenacious resilience, and recharged
by their determined commitment. Oftentimes we look at the won-
derful 'now' of a person's life without fully understanding the hell it
took to get there. **HOPE BEYOND FIBROIDS** *encompasses the*
full adventure...dipping you into the deepest valleys but lifting you
to unimaginable heights while reminding you... Never lose HOPE!"

—TeeJ Mercer
International Bestselling Author, Speaker, Reality TV Coach

"Everyone hopes for something. This was written for the women who
hope for children one day but keep hitting walls due to fibroids, infer-
tility, and other complications. Proverbs 13:12 says 'Hope deferred
makes the heart sick, but a dream fulfilled is a tree of life.' **HOPE**
BEYOND FIBROIDS *is about a dream fulfilled that is shared so*

that sick hearts can hope once more. Souls will be revived as they learn to hold on to what they have found to be elusive. My friend Gessie transparently shares the story of her journey to Nia and with authenticity becomes a tree of life for women pursuing their miracle babies. This book will have a profound impact on women who haven't found a place to share their pain, hopes, and prayers. Read it. Share it. Support it."

—Rev. Dr. Liz Rios | Founder, CEFL.Org &
Co-Pastor, Passion Christian Church

"I have had the opportunity to witness the decade-long journey Gessie Thompson traveled to childbirth. She was a model of grace and strength throughout. I have often, when faced with my own travails, asked myself 'What would Gessie do?' as a compass to navigate me through my storms. I'm sure **HOPE BEYOND FIBROIDS,** *and its collection of stories will become a compass for women going through similar issues and the men who love them."*

—Sharmayne Jenkins, Life Coach &
Adjunct Psychology Lecturer

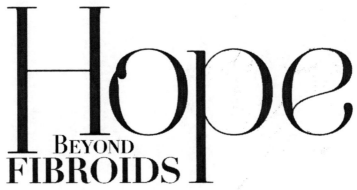

Hope
BEYOND FIBROIDS

*Stories of
Miracle Babies &
the Journey to
Motherhood*

GESSIE J. THOMPSON
with Coach Felicia T. Scott

nyreepress

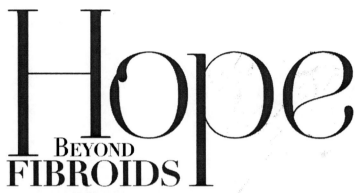

Hope

BEYOND FIBROIDS

*Stories of
Miracle Babies &
the Journey to
Motherhood*

www.HopeBeyondFibroids.com

HOPE BEYOND FIBROIDS
www. Hopebeyondfibroids.com
Copyright © 2015 – UpLift! Group
All rights reserved.

ISBN 978-0-9704898-3-8

Unless otherwise noted, Scripture quotations in this publication are from the New International Version (NIV), copyright © 1978 by New York International Bible Society.
Cover Designer: designBySpirit (www.designbyspirit.com)
Interior Designer: Jayleen Pepito (http://cuecodile.wix.com/jomel)
Photo Credit: All images have been used with the expressed permission of the contributor.
Photographer: Robert Fitch (www.robfitch.com)
Editor: Janet Hill Talbert
Editorial Assistant: Nicole L. Webb

Published by NyreePress Literary Group
Dallas, TX
www.nyreepress.com

For my husband and partner for life,
Marc, and our miracle, Nia—
you were worth every battle!

And to every prayer warrior who held up my arms in the
journey—there is no victory without obedience and faithfulness.

A special dedication to the late Dr. Myles & Pastor Ruth
Munroe—From the first time I heard you speak at Azusa and read
your book, "Understanding Your Potential," you taught me that I
was born on purpose, for a purpose, and with a purpose—one of the
very reasons we named our miracle baby Nia. My life has forever
been changed by the opportunity to learn from you, break bread with
you, and call you Papa Myles & Mama Ruth. Love you forever.

ACKNOWLEDGMENTS

arc—Thank you for being a godly leader, my friend, husband, coach, and greatest support. I can never thank you enough for our baby girl. I can't fathom our lives without her. I love you with HIS intensity and will continue to love you all the days of my life until death do us part. #ZaphenathPaneah

Nia—From inside my womb, you have taught me that only God has the right to determine our destinies. You defied every diagnosis and decided that no one could stop you from fulfilling your purpose. I am privileged to be your mother and praise God every day that He chose me for this high honor. #MamasBaby #OurMiracle

My Three Mothers—It's said that you can only have one mother, but I've been blessed with three! Thank you all for your tireless prayers and support every step in this journey. *Mom (Genevieve Jeanty)* – Without you I would not have life—physical or spiritual. Thank you for teaching me from birth to love the Lord. Your passion for Him ignited a desire in me to know and love Him from my youth and to continue to pursue Him daily. *Mama (Ezzie Scott)* – You taught me that love is thicker than blood and also the difference between a mother and a Mama. Thank you for adopting me as your daughter over thirty years ago and for loving me unconditionally as your own from day one. *Mommy (Cherral Jones)* – From the day we met, we were connected. Legally, you're my mother-in-law but we've always chosen Mother-In-Love to define our relationship. Thank you for loving me as your daughter rather than simply as your son's wife. #IWillAlwaysLoveMyMamas

My Three Dads—There are few relationships more impactful than a father to his daughter. *My Late Father (Richard Jeanty)*—You weren't perfect...but I'll love you forever, and I will always be your one and only Gessie. Your legacy of tenacity and passion lives on in your granddaughter, Nia and me. *My Late Daddy (Willie James Scott)*—Thank you for embracing me with open arms when I became an adopted member of the family and cherishing me as your own. Your golden heart and love changed me forever. *Pop Pop (John Jones)*—Nia's only living grandfather, you're a giant teddy bear with a big heart. From the day we met, you have loved, supported, and been there for me—helping whenever and however needed. Thank you! #FathersMatter

Nia's Biological & Spiritual Grand- and Great-grandparents—Adele Davis/Freddie & Virginia Gaston/ Jacques & Marie Gebara/Genevieve Jeanty/John & Cherral Jones/Ezzie Scott/Roslyn Abrams/Rose Andino/Connie Harris-Lennox/Pastor Katie Wright—Thank you for your tireless prayers, love, and support. #GenerationsofFaith

Felicia—My sister, coach, BFF, business partner, and coauthor! I can't thank God enough for bringing you into my life. He knows the purpose of our sisterhood, and I praise God for everything He has planned for us. #BFFLNMW

Naphtalie—For twenty-two years, I was an only child— and then came you. Every time I look at Nia, I see you. She's tenacious, feisty, bright, creative, and beautiful—just like you. #ABlackGirlWhoRocks

My Siblings—Jeannie/Andre/Carlos/Bernard & Nicole/ Brian & Thea/Taurean & Shawna/Emmanuel—As an only child for twenty-two (biological) years, I'm so grateful that God brought you into my life. #FamilyForever

My Godmother & Godfather—Yanick & Hantz Andre— Thank you for being an enduring example of a godly marriage! Your prayers, presence, and support over the course of my life, and especially during this journey, have been a gift from God. #GodlyLove

The Mingo Family—Denise—I am honored to count you as one of my dearest sister friends and blessed to have you as Nia's godmother. Your sisterhood challenges me to grow, motivates me to live, and inspires me to be better! *Alan*— Thank you for loving us and our Nia the way you do and for being a godly man that Nia can look up to as another model of Christ-likeness and manhood in her life. *Micah/Jordan/ Evan*—Thank you for being the best godsister and godbrothers that Nia could ever ask for. *My Spiritual Mother—MeMa*— You are a fierce prayer warrior, spiritual giant, Proverbs 31 woman, a Mama for the books, and a medical consultant to boot (LOL)! Thank you for praying for us without ceasing and for loving us the way you do. #TheMingosRock

My Family (Spiritual & Blood)—Jason & Esther/Crosby & Ellen/Dave T/David A & Alex/Nyasha/Charisse/Cornelius/ Mike & Regina/Derek & Cheryl/Cyril & Tyran/Scott & Tash/Tracey/Randy/Drew/Demo/Ray/Jonathan/Demo/KT/ Uncles, Aunts, Cousins—Your love, prayers, support, and friendship are daily helping me become the Gessie God purposed me to be. #FamilyByChoice

My Niece & Editorial Assistant—Nicole Webb—What a beautiful young woman you are inside and out! Thank you for your can-do attitude, awesome work ethic, inspiring optimism, commitment to excellence, beautiful spirit, and more. #MyNieceRocks

Janet Hill Talbert—My Friend & Editor—You didn't need to be bothered with my little project, but you accepted the assignment. Thank you for your friendship and for investing your gift in this vision. #RockStarEditorOnAssignment

ESSENCE Family—ESSENCE has always been the black woman's voice, champion, and advocate—giving platforms to issues that affect us deeply and uniquely. Thank you for shedding light on the fibroids epidemic that causes women of color to suffer in silence. #MyFertilityJourneyMay2014Page122

Tanika Gray Valbrun & The White Dress Project Board—Thank you for your friendship, partnership, and support in the fight against fibroids. #WeCanWearWhite #WhiteDressToTheWhiteHouse

Every Hope Beyond Fibroids Story—Thank you to every woman and man who trusted me to share your powerful testimony in this book of modern-day miracles. There IS #HopeBeyondFibroids

Special Thanks To—Pastor Samuels, Tricia (& the Woodstock Family) & Grafton, Sharmayne, Sharon & Brittany Webb, Kennisha Hill & NyreePress.

My Heavenly Father—You are the reason I live, and I'm so eternally blessed that You chose me. Thank You for everything You have brought me through and not allowing me to give up before You brought Nia into my life. I'm humbled that You chose me to be Nia's mommy, author this book, and play a role in the fight against fibroids; thank you for the grace to do it all to your glory. And please bless me to always remember that You are my greatest reward and to pursue You without abandon all the days of my life. #LovingYouIsMyPurpose

CONTENTS

BEYOND FIBROIDS

BEYOND THE EPIDEMIC

HOPE BEYOND FIBROIDS COACHING GUIDE EXCERPT WITH COACH FELICIA

FOREWORD

As a gynecologist, it is common for women to ask me about irregularities in their cycles. However, I find that many women are not aware of fibroids and how they can impact our lives. We spend so much time ensuring the well-being of others that we often neglect ourselves. When women have symptomatic fibroids, they often suffer in silence—waiting until things are unbearable before they choose to discuss them. Excessive bleeding, irregular cycles, severe cramping, and infertility become their "new normal."

In *HOPE BEYOND FIBROIDS: Stories of Miracle Babies & the Journey to Motherhood*, Gessie Thompson reveals a compelling account of her personal journey with fibroids as well as

the experiences of other women that she reached through sharing her story.

I love treating women and helping them with their journey
through reproductive life as well as into menopause. Fibroids
have become a large part of my practice—allowing me to discuss fibroid management with many women and offer surgical
options for some. When we look at the nature of fibroids, we
know that up to 70% of women have them by the age of 50 and
even higher for African American women—up to 80%!

The vast majority of fibroids are asymptomatic, and when
they do cause symptoms, it usually reveals itself with abnormal
uterine bleeding. The question then becomes, *What other symptoms are they causing and how do we deal with them?* Fibroids
can also cause pelvic pressure, infertility, bowel dysfunction, pain
with sexual intercourse, and bladder symptoms such as urinary
frequency and sometimes urgency.

As a woman with a daily front-row view of women dealing
with fibroids, I believe education will help them to understand
their bodies, their choices for treatment, and to ultimately feel
better. ***HOPE BEYOND FIBROIDS*** empowers women to
make more informed decisions through the experienced narrative of real-life triumphs and tragedies.

One of the most difficult impacts of fibroids to process is infertility. Fibroids can be found in 5-10% of infertile women. Based on the location of the fibroid, it can decrease fertility and hamper the ability to conceive. They can affect ovulation, fertilization, and implantation. And, the ensuing emotional ramifications of infertility can create a downward spiral that creates undue stress for both the women and her relationships.

After counseling women, I have watched their concerns snowball into anxiety, sadness, and, for some, depression. The quest for health when fibroids are involved requires well-trained and understanding physicians, informed patients, strong support systems, more research on preventative measures, and an assortment of treatments—including more breakthrough minimally invasive options—that will lead to successful outcomes.

This book addresses the questions of how women traverse their journey with fibroids and how THE *Hope Beyond Fibroids (faith)* can help women overcome their sometimes seemingly insurmountable obstacles. The observations and experiences that Gessie and the other women share are truly miraculous and astounding!

This moving collection of testimonies allows the struggle that women experience with fibroids to be shared among others through their own personal words and gives a point of view that is intimate and inspiring as you will see them persevere and eventually triumph. *HOPE BEYOND FIBROIDS* is unlike any other book, as it also addresses the questions many women have regarding their fibroids and also the expertise of medical doctors who are well versed in fibroids.

As a woman and a gynecologist who is passionate about helping women manage their fibroids, I am excited about Gessie's shared advocacy for creating large-scale awareness of this issue. The trials and triumphs in this book must be shared. Read on and allow *HOPE BEYOND FIBROIDS* to inspire you!

Dr. Jessica Shepherd MD, MBA
OB/GYN, Minimally Invasive
Trained Gynecologist
Founder of HerViewpoint.com

PREFACE

ind a mate. Get married. Add children to the family. As hard as the first two are, no one expects the third one to really be a challenge. At least I didn't... I know we didn't.

However, the "epidemic" of fibroids and ensuing infertility took Gessie and me on a fourteen-year odyssey through a myriad of emotions and experiences.

The inability to create new life with your wife is a challenge that rocks you to your very core as a man. It hits you squarely in your identity and forces you to come to terms with images and expectations that literally upend your sense of self.

Thankfully, through prayer, perseverance, and the God-given breakthroughs in medical science, the story of the Thompson family ends in triumph with a beautiful little girl, Nia Madison.

The human hero in this story is Gessie. The penultimate hero—as always—is a loving heavenly Father that sustained and supported her, and us, through it all with a community of family and friends.

You will read Gessie's story and those of other women, with a male perspective thrown in as well, and no matter where you are on your journey towards parenthood—looking forward with hope or reflecting backward in awe and wonder—you will be convinced forever that there is HOPE BEYOND FIBROIDS!

Marc Thompson, Jr.
Finance Executive,
Leadership Strategist &
Speaker (@MrUpLift)

INTRODUCTION

Growing up in church, I heard it so many times. "God will use your test to write your testimony, and your testimony will bless others." Or, said another way, "He's turning your mess into a message that will change lives." I saw this happen on a small scale in my everyday life. Providentially, I always encountered someone who needed the lessons I gleaned from something I'd just experienced. Little did I know that God in His omni-benevolence was weaving a testimony beyond my wildest imaginations through the "test" of my journey to motherhood.

In April of 2014, my life changed when my first-person narrative about my battle with fibroids was published in the May issue of *ESSENCE* and subsequently on the magazine's online and social media platforms. I was floored when "My Fertility

Journey" went viral on the iconic media outlet's Facebook page. My story was special to me, my husband, and family and friends, but never would I have dreamed that more than 33,000 people would like it on Facebook, with over 1,500 posting the story on their own timelines and 660 plus people commenting with their own miracle stories and thanking me for spreading hope by sharing mine.

And if that wasn't enough, I was invited to talk about it on other media platforms such as "The Tom Joyner Morning Show," "The Yolanda Adams Morning Show," "The Frank Ski Morning Show," ARISE TV, *Hope for Women* magazine, and more.

As a Talent Manager and Brand Strategist, my role is pitching the speaker or artist—not being the focus. So it was surreal to be on the other end of the camera and the subject of press materials. Yet and still, I yielded to and embraced God's sovereignty and determined that His plan for me was better than any plan I could imagine. I call it the Ephesians 3:20 blessing, which states, "Now to him who is able to do immeasurably more than all we ask or imagine, according to his power that is at work within us." (Ephesians 3:20)

As the calls, emails, Facebook messages, texts, and Twitter posts continued to roll in, it became clear to me that if my one story could have such a powerful impact on so many people, a book full of miracle stories could touch even more.

So I started to think about how I could best help women who were touched by my story and going through similar challenges. One day, my personal life coach and coauthor, Coach Felicia, asked me, "What did you need most when you were going through your journey?" My answer was clear. I needed hope.

As I continued to reflect on my struggle, I realized that my greatest enemy in the battle was not my fibroids, my surgeries, or even my infertility. It was hopelessness. If I could stay hopeful and encouraged, I could fight another day. On the days when my hope was broken, I would wither in defeat. And that's how the vision for this book was conceived. It would be a reference of testimonies called: *HOPE BEYOND FIBROIDS: Stories of Miracle Babies & the Journey to Motherhood.*

So I reached out on social media and requested stories from women everywhere, and people started to respond. As I read the litany of submissions, I saw the constant theme of God's miraculous hand in the lives of women on three paths.

First, there were stories of women who had miracle babies while battling fibroids—as I did—and had to navigate the infertility and/or pregnancy challenges that commonly arise as a result. Talking about the fibroids epidemic struck a resounding chord, as about 30% of all women will experience them by age thirty-five; and by age fifty, up to 60% Asian and Hispanic women, 70% of white women, and up to 80% of African American women will have fibroids—mostly affecting them during their reproductive years. Because of this, we've included, a section titled *"Fibroids FAQ with Dr. Cheruba Prabakar"* as well as a Glossary of Terms to help you navigate this prevalent women's health challenge. Dr. Cheruba was one of the doctors who cared for me during my two-month hospital stay.

Second, I noticed that there were women who suffered from non-fibroid-related infertility issues—stemming from complications such as endometriosis, an incompetent cervix, and more. Last, were stories of women who had no infertility issues but found themselves fighting for their babies due to complications that arose during pregnancy, post-delivery, or during the adoption process. Consequently, the book is divided into three sections to encourage women fighting for their miracle babies regardless of the circumstance: *Beyond Fibroids, Beyond Infertility,* and *Beyond Complications.*

If you are reading this book, I want to encourage you that God's plan for you is better than you can imagine (Ephesians

3:20). Trust in His good and perfect plan for your life (Jeremiah 29:11) and seek His will to set your priorities and direct your steps (Proverbs 3:5-7). If God has given you a vision for children and you are running into roadblocks, don't assume that means biological children. You may be spinning your wheels chasing after something when God has your child waiting for you through adoption. Conversely, if He has shown you that His plan for you includes biological children, hold onto His promise and never give up. No matter your situation—find your joy and peace in the gift of your relationship with God. No matter the disappointment or obstacle, let nothing separate you from His love (Romans 8:38). He is our greatest reward, and He is using this test to weave your testimony!

BEYOND FIBROIDS

Stories of women who had miracle babies while battling fibroids—as I did—and had to navigate the infertility and/or pregnancy challenges that commonly arise as a result.

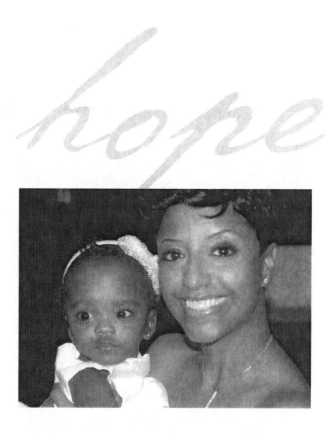

Hope In… The God Of Our Purpose

*"Many are the plans in a person's heart, but
it is the Lord's purpose that prevails."*

Proverbs 19:21

GESSIE THOMPSON

Never Quit... You Don't Know How Close You Are!

I became a first-time mother shortly after my fortieth birthday. On a beautiful September morning in 2011, Nia made her miraculous entrance into the world. I scarcely remember her first cry—and didn't even get to see her until the next day—because my heart stopped on the operating table as two world-class surgical teams worked to deliver her two-and-a-half-pound body. To this day, the doctors can't say exactly why it stopped, but one thing they all agree is that our Nia is nothing short of a miracle.

My journey to motherhood was a long and arduous one, beginning ten years earlier when my husband, Marc, and I decided we were ready to expand our family. But our plans were put on hold when a routine checkup revealed that I had uterine fibroids. I was vaguely familiar with them, as my mother had fibroids while pregnant with my younger sister, Naphtalie. She was told that Naphtalie would be deformed because a fibroid was pressing on her head—but Naphtalie miraculously defied the odds.

Knowing our desire to have children, my gynecologist (GYN) and I determined that an open myomectomy—an invasive surgery to remove the fibroids—provided the best opportunity to leave my uterus intact.

My surgery went well and recovery was textbook. My GYN at the time said that we should get pregnant within three to six months. Life went on, and though we desired to get pregnant, we weren't very proactive about it, believing that it would happen in God's time. Five years later, Marc and I still had no success conceiving. I knew something was wrong again when I began experiencing crippling abdominal pain, and making love became excruciating. The fibroids were back—with a vengeance.

Fearful of what this could mean to our dreams of parenthood, we consulted the highly recommended fertility specialists at the Center for Human Reproduction at North Shore LIJ. We discovered that the fibroids were so scattered in their placement that it would require an even more invasive surgery than the first time. Additionally, the fibroids were so big that my uterus spanned the size of a 15-week pregnancy! The doctor even commented that he didn't know how Marc and I were able to make love because one of the larger fibroids was sitting directly on my vaginal opening.

I'll never forget Dr. Rosenfeld's words: "It's going to be a difficult surgery and I'm going to have to cut you vertically in order to have the best chance at being successful." I immediately started bawling. The funny thing is that it was less about the fact that I had to have another surgery and more about his need to cut me from stem to stern. Please don't think me shallow, but for those few moments, all I could see was a nasty scar ruining my nearly perfect belly, and it was breaking my heart. *(Side Bar: Anyone who knows me is aware of my obsession with having a sexy belly.)* I apologized for seeming so silly and assured him that the most important thing was for him to do whatever he could to preserve my uterus.

I had my second myomectomy in 2006. It was a hard operation and an even more difficult recovery, which brought my first introduction to the nasogastric tube (NG). Dr. Rosenfeld explained that I had massive amounts of scar tissue from my first surgery. My recovery seemed to be going well, and I progressed according to schedule and went home within four days. However, I ended up going back and forth to the hospital several times because I wasn't able to keep food down. This concerned my doctors because this was a primary indicator that I might have developed a small intestine obstruction from the scar tissue.

Nine days after the operation, things had come to a head. I wasn't able to stop vomiting or eliminate any waste from my body. At the emergency room, a CT scan showed I had definitely developed an obstruction. Next would come my most horrid memory of every hospital stay in my journey. Hesitant to perform another surgery, the doctors put me on the NG tube because it would allow my digestive system an opportunity to rest and possibly decompress the obstruction by aspirating my stomach's contents.

I had to swallow down a tube as thick in circumference as my pinky by drinking a cup of water through a straw as the doctor inserted it through my nose, past my throat, and down into my stomach. I immediately developed a sore throat and could only communicate by writing on paper because it hurt too much to speak. I endured it all because my doctors felt it was my best chance at avoiding another surgery.

Unfortunately, it wasn't enough. Ten days after my second myomectomy and one of the most sleepless nights of my life, I found myself headed back into the operating room (OR) for a small intestine resection to remove the obstruction.

Recovery didn't get easier. I woke up, and the NG tube was still there—but it was no longer painful. I think it was because of the anesthesia and strong narcotics administered during the operation. Nonetheless, my battle continued as I quickly learned there were bigger issues for me to manage.

My surgeon informed me that the operation altered my digestive system, and it would take time for my body to create a new path to digesting food, drink, and even my own bodily fluids. I was designated NPO and could consume nothing by mouth until my digestive system showed evidence that it was activated again. The proof was passing gas. You might find this funny, but I've never prayed so hard to flatulate!

I was NPO for ten days and down to ninety-three pounds. I vividly remember the day it finally happened. I was beyond exhausted and walking the hospital corridors with my IV. Worship music was blasting in my ears through my iPod, and to ignite my faith I began walking around my IV seven times— fighting my own battle of Jericho. I knew my behavior may have seemed to strange to others, but I didn't care what anyone thought because I needed a breakthrough. I danced marching around that IV praising God. After I finished, I remember walking back to my room and passing the tiniest bubble of gas. I literally wept tears of joy for a biological process that was normally taken for granted.

After a total of twenty-one days in the hospital, I finally went home to complete my recovery and leave fibroids in my past.

At my first post-op exam, Dr. Rosenfeld explained to Marc and me that normal conception would be impossible for us going forward. There was too much scar tissue on my fallopian tubes and surrounding areas. Our only hope for getting pregnant would be In Vitro Fertilization (IVF). Undaunted, we got pregnant from my first IVF round in 2008. However, our hopes soon plummeted when our baby's heartbeat inexplicably stopped at week nine.

I can still recall every detail of that day as I walked out of the doctor's office into the hospital corridor after a special sonogram confirmed our deepest fears—we had miscarried at nine weeks. My legs were weak and I wanted to collapse, but Marc held me and said, "Not here, Baby." Referencing Scripture, he continued, "We don't grieve as those who have no hope." With every fiber in my body, I held it together until we got into our car, where we blasted Chris Tomlin's "How Great is our God" and "Holy is the Lord" while holding hands and crying our hearts out. We sang those profound lyrics at the top of our lungs, resolute that no matter how broken we felt in that moment, our God was GOOD and He was the only one who had the final say and He deserved our worship and adoration!

After grieving and healing, we tried two more IVF cycles in 2009 but were unsuccessful. Even more distressing was that all the while, the fibroids kept returning. In 2010, I endured a third myomectomy and second bowel resection. Hemorrhaging during surgery prevented the doctors from removing all the fibroids. My recovery was not as harsh as in 2006 but still long and slow, and I ended up in the hospital yet another twenty-plus days.

By this time I was thirty-nine and had a narrowing window of opportunity. We were racing against the fibroids for our dream. I was also wrestling with the effects of IVF and ready to give up. Physically, the medications were causing my vision to worsen, and the necessary hormone injections kept my emotions on edge, straining my marriage. I seemed to live in a state of anger, which made communication with me nearly impossible. In an effort to refrain from constantly reacting to my defensive tirades, Marc withdrew emotionally. I could tell that he was battling his own deep desire to become a father. He kept telling me that he would support whatever decision I made and to do what was best for me and my body. But I didn't want the responsibility of making the decision—I wanted him to tell me what to do!

Looking back, I thank God that Marc remained steadfast in encouraging me to hear from the Lord for myself. He gave me the gift of being able to stand resolute in my personal conviction that God was directing me to move forward with another round of IVF. Little did I know how much I would need that assurance in the near future.

Weighing the tension of past failed attempts and surgical complications against my husband's dream of biological fatherhood, I struggled to make a decision. I prayed for wisdom and direction and even secretly hoped the Lord would show us that His plan for us was not a biological child but adoption. But even in my struggle, I kept coming back to one prayer. "Lord, I am not my own, but I've been bought with a price. Your will be done in my life."

One morning I woke up and felt compelled to call my sister-friend Denise. We spent two hours on the phone, and she coached me with questions that helped me hear myself think. As I talked through it I had an "aha" moment that confirmed

Marc's words to me throughout this period. Now it was crystal clear. I saw that God had provided the way! For instance, for the first time our health insurance actually provided IVF coverage. Also, during my last surgery, the odds were against saving my uterus, but my doctor miraculously managed to do so. I felt confident that it was my time, and I was ready to try again.

A week later, my godmother Yanick called me. Though I hadn't shared my dilemma with her, she informed me that she'd stood in the gap for me during a special altar call for women who were trying to get pregnant. She told me that within a year I would have a baby. That confirming word became my faith's anchor!

We gave IVF one last try, and in February 2011, we got the call that we were pregnant!

But darkness loomed once more during a routine exam at twenty-one weeks when Dr. Rochelson, the Chief of Maternal Fetal Medicine at North Shore LIJ, discovered that our baby was severely underweight. An ultrasound revealed intermittent blood flow to the fetus, and I was diagnosed with Fetal Growth Restriction.

Stunned, my mother-in-love Cherral (aka Mommy), sister Felicia and I listened as he shared the textbook complications. My womb seemed destined to become a hostile environment. Words like "pre-term delivery" and "preeclampsia" landed like punches. And the words "We may want to talk about terminating the pregnancy" floored me.

Overwhelmed, I wanted to break down in tears in that moment, but I told him, "We are people of faith. And we believe in miracles." Dr. Rochelson responded, "I've been doing this long enough to know that everything can't be explained by medicine. So, buckle your seatbelt and let's ride it out."

I broke down in tears as I left the office. Ten years in, the fibroids were waging yet another war against me. They were leeches siphoning the blood supply our baby desperately needed. I had already been told a hysterectomy was imminent. This was our last chance! In that moment, we could have lost all hope, but our faith demanded we move forward. All I could hear was my godmother's voice telling me that I would have my baby in a year. It became clear that God gave me that word to sustain me during the storm that He knew would come. We were not giving up!

The next week, Marc and I met with Dr. Rochelson (he had been out of town on business during that initial visit and wanted to speak to the doctor directly). He listened as Dr. Rochelson explained everything he told us the week prior. Marc then asked, "Doctor, how long does my baby need to stay in the womb to be a healthy baby?" Dr. Rochelson responded, "Twenty-eight weeks." Marc rose up in faith and declared, "Doctor, my baby is going to give you between thirty-two and thirty-three weeks!" The doctor smiled and said, "Ok, Mr. Thompson." God was the only one with the final say so, and Marc and I were more determined than ever that we would stand in faith.

On Thursday, July 26, during yet another routine exam in my twenty-sixth week, an ultrasound showed that things had worsened and I was suffering from something called "reversal of blood flow." I was hospitalized immediately. Marc naively asked the nurse, "When will I be able to take my wife home?" She replied, "Mr. Thompson, we're just hoping the baby doesn't come before Monday." He then responded, "You don't have to worry. My son"—he thought we were having a boy—"will not be coming this weekend." We prayed for more time, and those three days turned into six miraculous weeks for our baby to grow!

Daily I endured a battery of nerve-wracking tests. But my husband, Mommy, and sister were always by my side. Having just started his first executive role at a fortune-10 company, Marc had just relocated from Queens to Schenectady, NY.

He drove home every weekend, coming straight to the hospital on Fridays after work. My two angels Mommy and Felicia split the day and night shifts—Mommy spending the days with me and Felicia the nights—supporting me through heart decelerations, emergency transports to labor and delivery, and more. Every day was a gift, and we had to be ready because it could have been the day that I was rushed to the OR for an emergency C-section.

Some time after the twenty-eighth week, on a Saturday morning during one of my daily sonograms, the attending doctor looked at me and said, "Mrs. Thompson, we didn't mean to scare you when you were first admitted, but in the textbook cases where reversal of blood flow occurs—such as in yours— the mother delivers within seventy-two hours. You're now at twenty-eight weeks, and we've never seen this before." I smiled and thanked God for His faithfulness.

God proved my husband's words to be true. On Tuesday, September 8, between thirty-two and thirty-three weeks, my doctors decided that the baby had a better chance in the world than in my womb and performed a C-section. The night before, the hospital allowed me to have my dream pregnancy photo shoot to document our miracle. I was overwhelmed by the reality of what the next day would bring. I was humbled by the dedication and kindness of the photographer, Robert Fitch, who worked with the administration and staff to turn my hospital room into a photo studio. There is no way to describe the serenity, because I truly felt like I'd found the sweet spot in God's hands and every joy in the world was mine.

At 10:50 a.m. on September 8, our miracle baby, Nia Madison Thompson, was born! She was underweight but in perfect health! She was feisty and all the nurses loved her. One told me, "I don't know who this little girl is going to be, but I hope I'm alive to see how she changes the world." We were able to take Nia home on Saturday, October 8, 2011—exactly one month after she was born. She now weighed 3 lbs 14 oz.

I'll never forget the ride home. As we pulled out of the hospital, Chris Tomlin's "How Great is our God" and "Holy is the Lord" were blasting in the car, but this time, we were crying tears of joy, shouting the lyrics at the top of our lungs.

The last time we left the hospital with those songs playing in the car, it was three years earlier and we had lost our baby to a miscarriage. This time we were driving home with a miracle.

God had kept His promise, and we were—and continue to be—immensely grateful! YES! Our God is GOOD, and He is the only one who has the final say and He deserves all our worship and adoration!

Today, Nia is three years old. She gives us immeasurable joy and daily lives up to the meaning of her name—purpose. Nia—she is a child born on purpose, for a purpose, and with a purpose.

Battling fibroids taught me to face facts with faith. We were covered in prayer by an army of family and friends. We're thankful for Drs. D. Rosenfeld, A. Hershlag, V. Klein, B. Rochelson, and the numerous doctors and nurses who respected our faith and their medicine.

Every day Nia reminds me to believe beyond my circumstances. My sister Coach Felicia says it best, "Never quit! You may know how far you've come, but you don't know how close you are!"

And My Journey Continued!

In 2012, after giving birth to Nia, I opted to treat my remaining fibroids with Uterine Artery Embolization (UAE). It was a simple and straightforward procedure. My follow-up examination showed that it was highly successful. I breathed a sigh of relief. I was forty-two years old and anticipated that menopause wouldn't be too far down the line and hormone changes would stop future fibroids from growing.

But as I worked to finish this book, I had to fight my final battle in the war to be #FibroidFreeForever! In early November 2014, I developed sinusitis and laryngitis. I felt miserable but didn't think I would be down for a long period of time.

Nearly three weeks later, on Saturday, November 29, 2014, my sister and I went to lunch after going to the hair salon. I was weak, lethargic, and I could tell something wasn't right. I said to her, "I feel like something is really wrong with me. I should be better by now, but I feel like I'm bleeding internally." Right away, she urged me to go the emergency room, and the next morning I did. In the ER, I complained of experiencing migraines every day, but a routine exam revealed that I had severe abdominal pain when the doctor pressed on my right side. I underwent both brain and abdominal CT scans, and while my head CT came back clean, my abdominal test showed two large fibroids— one pretty massive (tripled in size from the year prior).

I was in shock, and I felt like I'd been sucker punched! How could the fibroids have returned like this when I'd had the UAE procedure back in 2012? I thought for sure that procedure would tide me over until I started to go through menopause. I got ready to go home, and the nurse also gave me my lab results before heading out the door. I quickly scanned them and saw that my blood count showed my hemoglobin was down to an 8.2! No wonder I felt so listless. My hemoglobin level was six points below my norm of 14. I spoke to my God-brother who is a physician's assistant, and he told me that I was at levels normally found in post-surgical patients.

I called my primary care physician the next morning to find out what my blood count was on my last visit on Tuesday, November 11. My jaw dropped when the nurse shared with me that my hemoglobin on that day was 12.9! My mind wondered...how did I lose four units of blood in just under three weeks?

The following day, I called to schedule an appointment with Dr. Nimaroff, Chief of Gynecology at North Shore University Hospital. Miraculously, I was able to get an appointment that afternoon. The receptionist even said, "That spot must have been waiting just for you."

After examining and questioning me, Dr. Nimaroff informed me that the fibroids could not be the root cause of the blood loss I experienced. He suspected a gastrointestinal (GI) bleed. He also told me that the fibroids were very large, and I would need a hysterectomy because they should not have come back so aggressively after the UAE in 2012.

The next morning, I was scheduled to fly to Nassau, Bahamas, with my family for the memorial service of my mentors, Dr. Myles & Ruth Munroe. However, Dr. Nimaroff was concerned about my appearance and my extreme fatigue. He asked the nurse to draw more blood and check my hemoglobin level again. The results would determine whether or not he thought it was safe for me to travel.

The results came back, and in addition to feeling fatigued and extremely weak, I was now experiencing shortness of breath, tightness in my chest, and headaches. With a broken heart and much anguish, I finally relented; I would have to miss Mama Ruth and Papa Myles Munroe's service and get to the hematologist and gastroenterologist ASAP.

Two intravenous iron transfusions and a battery of five GI tests later—including an endoscopy, colonoscopy, capsule endoscopy, and two enteroscopies—the doctors finally got to the root cause of my drastic blood loss. The blood flow at the site of my first small intestine (or small bowel) resection had become compromised, and the tissue was severely ulcerated. This meant another major surgery—a complication clearly related to my previous fibroid surgeries! In addition to the hysterectomy, I would also need a small intestine resection.

I was desperate and fighting despair. After all the complications I'd had with my previous operations, the very last thing I wanted was to be cut again with not one but two major surgeries! My prayer warriors went to work and started sending me words of encouragement to strengthen my faith. I cast my cares on the Lord and resolved that He was the one ordering my steps. This meant I would rest in Him, trusting that He would "perfect that which concerned me" (Psalm 138:9).

On Monday, March 2, 2015, I underwent a seven-hour surgery to finally become fibroid free forever. My recovery was grueling and continues even as I write these words. After eighteen days filled with post-op complications—including low blood pressure; an elevated heart rate; a urinary tract infection; a yeast infection; never-ending level-10 pain that would only respond to heavy doses of IV Dilaudid (a narcotic pain medication) every three hours; multiple days of cramping diarrhea; severe uterine cramps that did not respond to any pain meds; a large collection of fluid; a drain inserted through my vagina and then another through my gluteus maximus, and last but not least, a setback that put me back on the NG tube—I am finally home recovering!

Every day in the hospital, it seemed there was another battle. And as I maintained my faith, the battles seemed to intensify. The last and most challenging test came two nights before I was discharged. After the second drain was inserted, my digestive system slowed down due to the general anesthesia and narcotics I had been taking for my unbearable pain.

After yet another CT-scan, I went back to my hospital room and vomited. I knew what this might mean, and my fears were confirmed by a physician's assistant who came to give me the results. She said, "Mrs. Thompson, the CT shows you've either developed an ileus or an obstruction, and if you continue to feel the way you do, we will have to put you on the NG tube to allow your digestive system to rest and hopefully heal." I screamed in my thoughts, "No...Not the NG tube! NO!!!" Her words threatened to break my spirit, and it took everything in me to hold it together.

It was nearly 2:00 a.m. and as the nausea intensified, two doctors and my nurse came in to insert the tube from hell. Thank God for my sister who was with me and kept reassuring me that it was going to be all right. The tube was in, and every time I swallowed it kicked the back of my throat like a soccer ball. Finally a peaceful sleep came over me and allowed me to rest for a few hours.

About 6:00 a.m. I woke up and immediately went out into the corridor to walk and pray.

From my previous experience with the NG tube, I knew that it couldn't be taken out until my digestive system was reactivated and I passed gas. My faith was on trial, and I was not going to lose this battle. I remembered my victory back in 2006 and decided I would walk around seven times again. As I walked, I spoke the Word over my life and my circumstances. With every breath in my body, I affirmed, "God, it doesn't matter what I feel right now. I know that your Word is true and you exalt your Word above your name. You watch over it to perform it, and I thank you that by the stripes of Jesus I am healed. I command my digestive system to be alive and active, working perfectly. Body, you will come in line with the Word of God and operate according to the perfection to which God created you to function."

After my seventh time around, I walked back into my room and rested in the chair beside the bed. About thirty minutes later, I felt my body release gas twice! I jumped up, clapping my hands and shouting, "Hallelujah, hallelujah, hallelujah!!! Thank you, Lord!" I called for the nurse and had her update the doctors immediately so they could take the tube out. The next evening, I was finally released to go home!

Before I went into the hospital, I asked everyone to pray with me that I would have an easy and quick recovery. That is the antithesis of what I experienced. But the Lord reminded me the other day that everyone wants to be a winner but there is no victory without a battle! My fibroids were the cause of every challenge I faced on my journey to motherhood—physical and spiritual. They waged war against me, my baby, my marriage, and my purpose! But by God's grace I am victorious; I am the winner. I am the mother of the amazing Nia Madison Thompson. I am now finally #FibroidFreeForever, and this book, *HOPE BEYOND FIBROIDS*, my spiritual baby, has been born! To God be **ALL** the glory!!!

hope

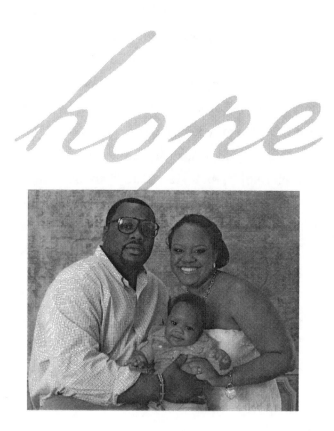

Hope In… The God Who Answers

"I prayed for this child, and the Lord has granted me what I asked of Him."

1 Samuel 1:27

KAZMIR DAVIS

God Can. God Will. God Did!

My journey to motherhood began long before I was in position to really become a mother. While we were dating, my husband, Terrence, used to refer to me as an "MIT"—"Mother in Training"—because I was always caring for someone else's child. Nine months into our marriage, I shared with my husband the news that we were expecting. We hadn't planned it, but we hadn't taken precautions to avoid it either.

I was so excited that I immediately started registering on baby websites and making changes to my diet. From the moment I saw that double pink line on the pregnancy test, I began making moves to ensure I was "doing everything right" for my baby.

Our exciting journey soon became a stressful one when our midwife could not detect a heartbeat during our second prenatal appointment. My heart dropped, but the midwife encouraged us to not worry because, "This happens all the time. It may be too early to find the heartbeat, or the little one could be hiding in there," were the words she used to help calm our fears. The following day, we were scheduled for an ultrasound screening for fetal heart tones.

We quietly left the office, and as soon as I closed the car door, I burst into tears. I went home, climbed in bed, and saturated my pillow as I cried out to God, praying that everything would be all right. My husband comforted me throughout the night, but my heart remained unsettled.

The next day, an excruciating eighteen hours later, we were told that my ultrasound appointment would have to be pushed off another two weeks because of healthcare politics. There was no way my nerves could take another two weeks of waiting, so at my husband's suggestion, we decided to go to the emergency room.

It was in the ER on July 12, 2011, that I heard those unforgettable words—"I'm sorry, the baby did not survive."

Those words literally KNOCKED THE WIND OUT OF MY CHEST!

I was informed that I'd had what's called a missed abortion. I'd miscarried, but my body wasn't yet aware and was still functioning as if I was pregnant. This was also the first time I learned that I had several fibroids, which played a significant role in my losing the baby. I endured a Dilation and Curettage (D&C) procedure and left the hospital empty.

I was devastated by the loss of our baby. I questioned, "God, why me?" It wasn't fair! I thought I had done everything right! I had saved myself for marriage and changed my diet to preserve my health for the pregnancy. Even more painful was the fact that all the women in my life were getting pregnant. I couldn't help but wonder if there was something wrong with me as a woman.

Terrence was very supportive, but our loss took an emotional toll on our marriage. My grief was so overwhelming and consuming that he began to feel as if I wanted to be a mother more than I wanted to be his wife. Thankfully, we kept the door of communication open, and with coaching from our pastor and faith in God, our marriage survived the storm. In that season, I learned what scripture means when it says,

GESSIE J. THOMPSON *with*

COACH FELICIA T. SCOTT

"All things work together for the good" (Romans 8:28). My confession was, "Since things aren't good in this moment, God is not done!"

Some time later, I was introduced to an amazing and anointed obstetrician, Dr. Deslyn Mancini, who declared, "God is a BIG God...He is in control; don't worry."

From the moment I walked into her office, I could feel the presence of God resting in the atmosphere. I felt safe under her medical care and trusted that God would, in fact, bless us indeed. Dr. Mancini initiated the efforts to have the fibroids removed, and on July 12, 2012, exactly one year after losing my baby, I had a robotic myomectomy.

After a successful surgery, my husband and I were actively trying to conceive. And once again while we were in the midst of a challenge, everyone around us was getting pregnant or having babies. Secretly, there were moments when those baby bumps taunted me. Outwardly, I had to put on a smile, and even though I was sincerely happy for others, I could not help but wonder, "When will it be our time?"

I know why Hannah in the Bible cried! There was a civil war going on inside me—a fight to believe when my eyes couldn't see. I had to trust that God was working on our behalf, but it seemed like nothing was going on! Every twenty-eight days, I was on a crazy emotional roller-coaster ride and would vacillate between faith and despair! I was either emotionally numb or hysterical!

In May 2013, during my annual exam with Dr. Mancini, she told me that it was good that I hadn't gotten pregnant yet. She preferred a one-year recovery period from my myomectomy surgery. Her exact words again were, "God knows what He is doing. He is a BIG God! He is in control!"

I left the appointment that day with a peace I have never felt before. This was the first time since my miscarriage that I truly felt submitted to the will of God for my life. I was at peace with it all and so grateful for Dr. Mancini, a physician of strong faith and conviction, and that she had spoken so powerfully into my life about my situation.

My husband and I were content in knowing God could do it! That very fact allowed me to rest on His promises and not stress about whether or not we were pregnant. I was satisfied in knowing "GOD CAN!"

Our spiritual father, Pastor Troy Davis, was also led to speak into my life that my womb was ready and began to pray for a full-term, healthy, and strong pregnancy. Dr. Mancini vowed to continue to intercede on our behalf and told us to get two other intercessors to start praying and suggested "Mother White" from our church.

That next Sunday, we spoke with Rev. Marie White and Evangelist Theresa Lyons—two intercessors at our church—and solicited their prayers. Evangelist Lyons declared in that instant, "GOD CAN and GOD WILL!"

The next few weeks were spent in sheer bliss with my husband. We were enjoying life and felt totally confident in God's ability to bless us in His time.

On July 12, 2013—exactly two years to the date of our first miscarriage—God did it. We were pregnant again! The joy that flooded my soul was indescribable! To experience a hand-of-God miracle was astounding and breathtaking.

On March 13, 2014, I went into labor. We filled the atmosphere with worship, playing Israel and New Breed's Pandora station, yet there was a balance between calm and anxiety. Right before I was ready to deliver the baby, his heart rate dropped tremendously. But as William Murphy's "Let It Rise" played, we began to pray and break out into worship. God was truly in the midst of it all!

Zion Isaiah Davis, our miracle baby, weighed 8 lbs and 3 oz and was welcomed into the world via a Cesarean section because of my previous myomectomy. The moment I heard him cry, I cried out to God with the voice of triumph. As soon as the doctors put him near me, he reached out and touched my face, assuring me that he was responsive. My heart remembered the scripture "For this child I prayed, and the Lord has granted me what I asked of Him" (1 Samuel 1:27).

Zion Isaiah is truly a miracle and brings so much joy to our family. His smile makes my heart melt and continues to remind me that God is able to do "exceedingly, abundantly, above all we can ask or think, according to the power that works in us" (Ephesians 3:20). What we thought was a tragedy was really an opportunity to experience God like we had never experienced Him before. God Can! God Will! God Did!

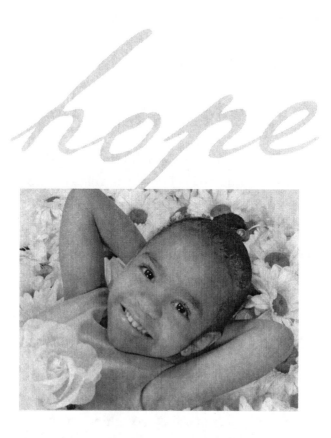

Hope In... The God of Unfailing Love

"The Lord delights in those who fear him,
who put their hope in his unfailing love."

Psalm 147:11

PERDITA CHAVIS

My Baby, Miracle

"Yep, you're pregnant, Ms. Chavis," Dr. Prater assured.

He continued sifting through my file, a thick sheaf of papers containing diagnoses over the past twenty years. He had just officially confirmed what a home test revealed earlier in the week. I sat on the examining table, bewildered and grateful that I had worn my winter jacket, as an inexplicable chill spread over my body. I shivered—unsure if it was the cold office or nervousness. My mind was a whirlwind of questions, but my thoughts were interrupted by a frown that began to spread across Dr. Prater's forehead.

Three years before in August 1999, at Dr. Prater's urging, I underwent surgery to remove extremely painful fibroid tumors. What was supposed to be a simple three-hour surgery to extract seven tumors turned into a twelve-hour surgery to take out thirteen!

Although my recovery went well, the prognosis was not optimistic. During one of my follow-up visits, Dr. Prater explained that the chance of more fibroids growing and multiplying still existed, therefore lessening the possibility of me ever carrying a child full term. I had taken his prognosis lightly, because at the time I was a recently divorced thirty-seven-year-old, and the thought of becoming a parent was the furthest thing from my mind. I was enjoying my career and my life. Then, in late October 1999, I met Marco.

Marco was a handsome man, a few years my senior, with dark, short curly hair, caramel skin tone, and a sultry voice to boot. We connected instantly. We enjoyed doing the same things, eating the same foods, and loved the same music. Our casual dating gradually progressed into a committed relationship. We traveled together and sailed on two cruises in a year. It was during that last cruise that I believe I conceived. The moment I stepped off that ship—I knew. My body told me its secret. My insides crashed around like the waves of the ocean—constantly hitting me as if I was on the shore.

As I sat on the examining table, Dr. Prater reminded me of the prognosis from 1999. He cautioned me that my pregnancy might not continue full-term because my new fibroids could potentially threaten the growth of my baby. I sat staring at Dr. Prater, and a lone tear streamed slowly down my face. Yet he was optimistic and suggested my pregnancy be monitored through a series of sonograms at least once or twice a month. I agreed and left Dr. Prater's office.

As I walked to my car the words "threaten the growth of the baby" kept repeating over and over in my head. I reached my car and sat in the driver's seat for what seemed like hours. I wondered, "I God punishing me for conceiving my baby in sin?" So, I prayed and accepted God's will. I felt a calm wash over me then started my car and drove home.

Later that evening at home, I debated about telling Marco about my pregnancy over the phone or face-to-face. I decided to tell him in person, but then my telephone rang—he was calling me! We chatted casually for a few minutes, asking about each other's day, and then I said, "I have something to tell you."

"You're pregnant," he blurted, and I sat there holding the phone in amazement.

"What made you say that?" I asked. "How did you know?" He replied that he'd had a feeling. When I asked him how he felt, he said he was both uncertain and elated at the same time. I told Marco Dr. Prater's concerns about the pregnancy, and he said, "Well, we have to leave this in God's hands." I agreed and again experienced a feeling of calm.

I endured the monthly sonograms at an imaging center, not eagerly, nor happily, but obediently. I sometimes griped, but the griping ceased after the fifth sonogram. During one visit, I was watching the monitor as the sonogram technician moved the wand across my growing belly. On the monitor, I could vaguely determine the shape of a little person, unsure at the time if it was a girl or a boy. I narrowed my eyes and continued looking at the monitor, in an effort to decipher the round shape that was adjacent to that little person. "Is that another little person?" I asked the sonogram technician. Her only response was, "Your doctor will answer any questions you have."

I was so eager to meet with Dr. Prater; my appointment for the following week could not come soon enough. I wobbled into his office with Marco beside me, walking with his arms outstretched and ready to catch me in case I fell. Eagerness overwhelmed me, and I think Dr. Prater sensed it, for he wasted no time with the results from the sonogram. The round shape that I saw adjacent to my little person was a fibroid tumor. It turned out that it was growing with my baby and was actually pushing my baby out of my womb. I was devastated!

Marco hugged me tightly, and as he did, I could feel his body trembling against mine. He kept reassuring me that everything was going to be okay, but I think his words were for not only me but for himself as well. Dr. Prater offered words of encouragement and suggested more frequent sonograms; Marco and I agreed.

After we left the doctor's office, Marco and I prayed in his truck—we prayed for our baby and for God's will. As we exited the parking garage, I felt a new feeling of warmth and calm overwhelm me. I could not understand the peace that came upon me, and even though I knew that the fibroid was jeopardizing the growth of my baby, I proclaimed and accepted God's will.

As I arrived home, everything Dr. Prater said continued to run through my mind, and I began crying out to the Lord. I asked God for forgiveness—I knew that I had sinned in conceiving my baby out of wedlock. I felt ashamed because

I wanted so badly to be an obedient servant, yet I had succumbed to temptation more than once. I'm sure this was why I thought that I was being "punished." I prayed to God to spare my baby's life and not hold my sins against him/her. I guess one might say that I made a deal with God, even though I know that He's not in the dealing business but the blessing business. I talked to God and told Him that although I had fallen short, I was still a willing servant.

It wasn't easy, but I knew I had the prayers and support of my family. They prayed together monthly—many generations would gather together and intercede for my baby and me.

A couple of months after receiving the news of the fibroid's attempt to take over my womb, my mother called for a special family prayer. Many of my family members—approximately thirty of us—gathered in my mother's den. We prayed for Marco, our baby, Dr. Prater, and me. After prayer, we feasted on my mother's gumbo!

Another month passed, and I reached the eighth month of my pregnancy. On the day of my next-to-the-last sonogram, Marco drove me to the imaging facility for my appointment. It was old hat to me by then, so I laid down on the examining table and watched the sonogram monitor. I could see that my baby was growing and looked more like a little person. The sonogram technician asked if we wanted to know the sex of the baby. I at first replied, "No!" yet quickly changed my mind, and Marco and I stated in unison, "Yes!" The sonogram technician told us our little person was a girl.

At that moment, I saw pink ballerinas dancing in my head, but the dancing was cut short when I noticed the look on the face of the sonogram technician. I watched as she repeatedly moved the sonogram wand across my belly. She repeated this movement over and over, yet when I asked for a reason she declined, stating that my doctor would review everything with me. "Oh boy, here we go again," I thought.

The next week, Marco and I went in for our appointment to review the sonogram results with Dr. Prater. As we waited to see him, we had already resolved to be strong. I had accepted that I may not be able to carry our baby girl full-term, but I was grateful for the experience. I needed to tell myself something to maintain my sanity!

Dr. Prater called us into his office and offered us seats. I could not help but focus on his desk, which was a large, old pecan wood, rectangular structure with a thick glass top. Underneath the glass were hundreds of photos of various sizes. They were pictures of newborns and toddlers that Dr. Prater had delivered. I longed to have a photo of my baby girl displayed in that collage!

Dr. Prater's voice brought me back to reality as he stated he wanted to discuss the results of the sonogram. He told us that he had ordered another one to be conducted in his office in order to confirm the results of the last sonogram.

Marco and I were puzzled. Dr. Prater then explained that the last sonogram did not detect the fibroid that had been growing with our baby girl. He stated that it had possibly shrunk. Marco and I were thrilled and looked at each other with excitement and hope.

The results of the new sonogram seemed to take forever! While we waited, Marco and I prayed. I telephoned my mother with the hopeful news and asked her to call the rest of the family, and she obliged. Dr. Prater finally called Marco and I into his office again. As we took our seats, I focused again on Dr. Prater's desk! This time I was searching for the spot where our daughter's picture would be displayed.

Dr. Prater confirmed our hopes. The second sonogram indicated that the fibroid tumor had indeed shrunk! Marco and I both cried tears of joy and thanksgiving. Dr. Prater offered us congratulations and advised me to begin taking leave from work because the latter part of my term was critical.

We practically skipped to Marco's truck. My huge belly made my version awkward and wobbly, but I didn't care! I wanted everyone to know and feel my joy—our joy! We could not wait to share the news with our other family members. Everyone was elated and began making plans for the baby's arrival.

Marco and I were so consumed with the ordeal of whether or not I would carry the baby to full term that we had not thought of a name. One night, as I lay in bed, I thanked God over and over, and I committed our baby girl to God. I prayed that His will be done in her life.

As I concluded my prayer, I heard the word "Miracle" in a whisper. I looked around, searching for the source to no avail. However, I continued to hear Miracle repeatedly in my head and in my heart. "That's it," I yelled. "We will name our baby girl Miracle, for she is God's miracle to us!" I called Marco right away. "Miracle—her name will be Miracle, for she is that," I said. "Wonderful! That's perfect," Marco replied.

On a hot afternoon in late July 2003, our Miracle arrived two weeks earlier than expected. Most members of my immediate family were present, causing the nurses to joke that they had never seen a delivery room full of so many people. Miracle came into this world and into our lives despite the threat of that fibroid tumor.

A few days after Miracle and I came home from the hospital, I sat in my soft, dark gray living room chair holding her in solitude, in awe of the wonders of God. I reflected on how He allowed me to bring this beautiful human being into the world. I knew then that I needed to become fully obedient to God and live according to His will. I made a commitment to God that I would be His vessel, and I rededicated myself afresh to Him. I vowed celibacy, partly out of fear, for I did not want to disappoint God, and of course, because I wanted to submit to Him.

Today, Miracle is a smart and talented eleven-year-old with a beautiful spirit and a genuine heart. She loves to hear me tell the story of how we came to name her, and I never miss the opportunity to tell her how God's grace is so amazing!

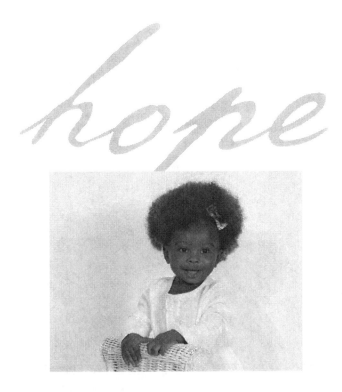

Hope In... The God Who Gives Life

"I shall not die, but live, and declare the works of the LORD."

Psalm 118:17 KJV

JOCELYN
GOODING-SMITH

You Shall Live!

My husband, Curtis, and I had been happily married for ten years, and people always commented on our relationship—*I wish I had what you guys have! You guys are a match made in heaven! Have you considered joining the Family Life Ministry at church?* These are just a few of the comments that we often heard—and thankfully still do. However, there were other comments and questions that we couldn't answer—*When are you guys going to have kids? Don't you want children? How come you guys don't have children?*

Honestly, these questions were extremely painful for us because only we knew what was happening behind the scenes.

We had been trying and trying and trying to conceive. There were times when we thought we were close to having our dreams realized, but I ended up having several miscarriages.

We didn't know where to turn, because infertility is not something that is discussed openly in the church. In our case, it wasn't because our church was against dealing with sensitive issues. It's just that nobody was talking about it! We were getting our spiritual and emotional needs met in church… but who wants to stand up and admit that they have this problem? In hindsight, we realize that maybe we should've been the ones to speak. Regardless, I am eternally grateful for the prayers and support our pastors, Dr. Roderick and Rev. Beverly Caesar, offered as we endured each miscarriage.

I believe our journey to becoming parents was filled with miracles. The first one happened on the night of our last miscarriage; we met Dr. Victor Klein of North Shore University Hospital (NSUH). He is one of the most sought-after high-risk pregnancy obstetricians in the country and has appeared on *Oprah* and other acclaimed TV shows. After treating us that night, he sent us to a well-known fertility specialist, Dr. Gabriel San Roman.

Sitting with Dr. San Roman was eye-opening. The first thing he told us was that he was just a vessel used by "The Man Upstairs," and it was God who would bless us with a child. How fitting given our Christian values! The next thing he talked about was the treatment that we would both need. The costs connected to these procedures were astronomical, but God had a plan.

We were entered into a very small study and, as a result, all of our medical expenses were covered. Every procedure, every medication, every sonogram, EVERYTHING was covered at no cost to us! I count that as miracle number two.

After several rounds of artificial insemination, we moved on to In-Vitro Fertilization (IVF). After two rounds and twelve failed eggs later, on the day the study closed, we got pregnant with the final egg!

The pregnancy proved to be very difficult. On January 19, 2011, I was told that I was having a full-blown miscarriage and bled for three days. I vividly remember that day—I started bleeding at work, and my boss called my husband. Curtis called the doctor, who told us to come right in. By the time we arrived, my clothes were soaked. I was losing blood, hope, and faith.

My husband encouraged me to believe that God promised us this child, and I clung to his faith. Having a husband who believes the Lord when you cannot is a true blessing. The nursing staff told us that things did not look good but that they were going to look for a heartbeat. Sure enough, there it was! There was still life inside, and we could hear it! However, the blood was coming from a huge hole in my uterus. We prayed desperately for a miracle.

Within three days, the hole was gone. All of the staff was stunned, as they had not experienced anything like this before. With that, we continued on our journey of becoming parents. Yet, another miracle—number three!

The next few months were challenging, to say the least. I remained on bed rest for six months because I was in active labor. I had fibroids that were crowding our baby girl— pushing her out of the womb. I was having full-blown contractions, and they were painful. Can you imagine being in labor for six months? I spent more time in the hospital then out. The pain was unbearable. The magnesium I was on to stop the contractions actually made me sick.

The doctors thought that Kaitlyn would be premature and believed that she would be born at twenty-two weeks. I was constantly in and out of the hospital. It felt like I was Norm from the old television show *Cheers*. Everyone knew my name and greeted me accordingly.

My obstetrician, Dr. Klein, ruled out a natural delivery for me because of the fibroids and told me I had to have a C-Section. I was also told I needed to have a special surgeon who dealt with high-risk deliveries in the room since the procedure was risky but he was unavailable to perform my surgery. Dr. Klein quickly called one of his close colleagues, Dr. Andrew Menzin, to my rescue. Dr. Menzin is a gynecological surgeon, but he is also the Associate Chief Gynecology Oncology of Obstetrics & Gynecology at NSUH. He was heading home when he got the call, but praise God, Dr. Menzin agreed to come and perform the procedure. My C-Section began as soon as he arrived— miracle number four!

Our daughter, Kaitlyn, was born full-term on August 23, 2011—the day of the East Coast Earthquake! You would never know the struggle she endured in utero! The only physical evidence is a slight indentation on her forehead where one of the fibroids pushed against it while in the womb. She spent five days in the hospital's Neonatal Intensive Care Unit (NICU) so that doctors could monitor her. She was released on August 28, 2011, the day Hurricane Irene struck New York—talk about taking the world by storm! But she was here—miracle number five!

Upon opening me up, the doctors found numerous fibroids, but there was one in particular that especially concerned Dr. Menzin. Weeks later we would find out that his suspicions were well founded. It turned out that within one of the fibroids was a very rare and aggressive cancer sarcoma, also called a leiomyosarcoma. In more than 99% of fibroid cases, the tumors are benign.

The cancer would not have been discovered had it not been for the Cesarean Section. Normally, by the time this kind of cancer is discovered, it's usually too late. I was told that my chances for survival were very slim and was given five years to live.

Three years after my initial diagnosis and three reoccurrences later, I am still here and believing that God has another miracle on deck for me. I choose to believe that by Christ's stripes, I am healed. Miracle number six!

After taking my daughter home, we had several more tests of faith to endure. She had trouble moving her bowels.

The doctors couldn't understand the root cause of this issue. One night as my husband held her, he prayed over her and commanded her bowels to move… and they did!

In May 2014, during a surgical procedure, Kaitlyn simply stopped breathing while on the table. They worked on her while my husband, friends, family, pastor, and I went to chapel to pray. Two-and-a-half hours later, Kaitlyn was on a respirator and remained in an induced coma for a week. Thankfully, she recovered and there is no evidence of any long-term or residual challenges

Today, my daughter is a healthy, happy, bright, talented three-year-old, and because sarcoma is not a blood disease, she was left unaffected by the cancerous fibroid.

I recently became a minister at Bethel Gospel Tabernacle and have had the opportunity to talk about a subject that is near and dear to my heart—infertility. My husband and I are still in love with God and each other, and we believe that He is still in the miracle-working business. "I shall not die, but live, and declare the works of the LORD" (Psalm 118:17).

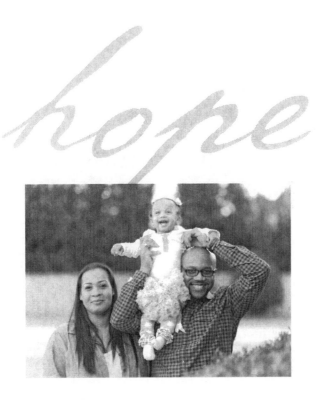

Hope In... The God Of Our Dreams

*"'For I know the plans I have for you,'
declares the LORD, 'plans to prosper you and
not to harm you, plans to give you
hope and a future.'"*

Jeremiah 29:11

NIA CLEVELAND

My "I Have A DREAM" Baby

was born to be a mother. Even as a child, I dreamed of having children of my own. Nurturing and caring for others comes naturally to me. Ask anyone who knows me, and they will tell you that I'm the mothering type. But even though my maternal instinct was a "no-brainer" in my heart, my body didn't agree.

In 2003, I was diagnosed with uterine fibroids. Originally, I had mixed emotions. On one hand, I was really nervous because I knew this could possibly mean surgery in the future. On the other hand, I'd watched my mother and three sisters live with fibroids, so it wasn't something rare or unusual. My doctor's advised me to "leave them alone" unless they started to bother me…but bother me they did!

I started experiencing the classic telltale symptoms: heavy bleeding, breakthrough bleeding, and cramping. At its worst, my menstrual cycles lasted around nineteen days each month. The almost constant bleeding left me severely anemic, and I would often feel dizzy and faint. I couldn't deny it—surgery was imminent!

Two years later, in the summer of 2005, I had my first myomectomy. I quickly recovered and felt like a brand-new woman! For me, uterine fibroids were a thing of the past. But in 2010, I started experiencing familiar and distressing symptoms. The fibroids were back!

But it was different this time around...Now I was a thirty-year-old newlywed. My husband, Alvin, and I were eager to start our family right away. The fibroids loomed like a threat to our fragile dreams.

I expressed my concerns to my doctor, and she prescribed Lysteda—a drug that would help control my bleeding without interfering with my fertility. My husband and I tried for an entire year and did not conceive. Consequently, my doctor referred me to a fertility specialist. Although I wasn't overjoyed at the prospect, I was still hopeful and optimistic for my future family.

The fertility specialist sent me to get an MRI of the fibroids to assess my situation and pinpoint the root of my fertility complications. After reviewing my results, he recommended that the fibroids be removed. We discussed several different treatment options: a classic myomectomy, UFE (uterine fibroid embolization), and a hysterscopic myomectomy. We came up with a complicated surgery plan, using UFE for my large fibroid and a hysterscopic myomectomy for the smaller two. In an effort to shrink my fibroids before surgery, he prescribed Lupron to temporarily send my body into early menopause.

At the end of the surgical consultation, I made the mistake of asking the specialist what advice he would give his daughter if she were in my position. He didn't miss a beat and replied, "I'd tell her to adopt."

His words shattered my faith like a brick flying through glass. They played in my head over and over...torturing my heart. I literally felt hope leave my body every time I recalled the doctor's comments. But I still had a mustard seed grain of faith left—I was not giving up!

Depressed and heavyhearted, I called my older sister and told her about the conversation. Upon hearing the specialist's reply to my last question, she caught an attitude and told me point blank, "I don't like that doctor!" I thought to myself, "Me neither!"

At that moment, I decided I wasn't comfortable with him. My sister suggested that I go to Chicago and meet with her OB/GYN, Dr. John Hobbs, who was also an ordained minister. I had nothing to lose, so I took an unconventional approach and wrote him letter explaining my situation. I told Dr. Hobbs that my husband and I desperately wanted to start our family, and I wanted to do everything possible to preserve my fertility.

To my surprise, after receiving my letter, Dr. Hobbs called me! He said that my words tugged at his heart and that he and his colleague would love to help me. I instantly felt a sense of peace and made the decision to switch doctors and travel to Chicago for the surgery.

In July of 2012, I took a month-long medical leave from work and had my second myomectomy, which proved to be far more complicated than expected. I'd developed massive amounts of scar tissue around my intestines from my first surgery.

After my recovery, the physician told me to wait three months and then "go make a baby!" My husband and I waited, and in three months, we got to work on following the doctor's orders.

Still...no baby was made. But I was optimistic because I knew from all the literature I'd read that "making a baby" could take around six months.

One day while driving, I noticed an oddly placed fertility clinic. I wrote down the name and Googled it when I got home. I decided to contact them to set up an appointment. There I met Dr. Barry Ripps, who did a thorough work-up. I was heartbroken when he discovered yet another fibroid that needed to be removed. It was now early 2013.

I felt defeated, angry, and frustrated. I was fed up with fibroid surgeries. The doctor explained that he could remove this new fibroid tumor with a minimally invasive laparoscopic surgery and it would be an outpatient procedure. It went well, but we discovered a new medical obstacle in the process. My fallopian tubes were covered with scar tissue. This was contributing to my infertility and would have put me at risk for an ectopic pregnancy. During the laparoscopic procedure to remove the new fibroid, he cut away as much scar tissue as he could to optimize my chances at conceiving and having a healthy pregnancy. However, significant scarring remained, so he recommended that Alvin and I try In-Vitro Fertilization (IVF) as our best option.

Two weeks after my laparoscopic procedure, I was given the green light to start fertility treatments! I started classes at the clinic to learn how to inject myself with the IVF medications. It was scary at first, but I was ready to do whatever it took to become a mother.

At the end of one of my classes, my doctor mentioned that he wanted to do a follow-up exam to check on my progress from the laparoscopic surgery. After the examination, he informed me that there was now another fibroid inside my uterus that needed to be removed. I was given the option to move on with the treatment without the surgery but was advised that leaving the fibroid could negatively affect the implantation of the embryo.

I felt absolutely depleted and defeated as I lay on the examination table...once again discussing my options. I didn't want another surgery or procedure. I just wanted to have a baby! Like any other mother, I wanted the best future for my baby. My desire for a healthy baby was greater than my apprehension and dismay—I decided to have the surgery.

Everything went perfectly in surgery, and I was able to start fertility treatments soon after. We hit the jackpot after my first round of IVF. I was pregnant with twins! We found out during my sixteenth week that the babies were girls. Alvin and I were elated! All of the heartaches, the tears, and the prayers were worth it. I had the most important job in the world—carrying my babies!

Due to my surgical history and the fact that I was carrying twins, my pregnancy was classified as "high risk," so I was scheduled to see my doctor weekly. During an examination at my seventeen-week appointment, the doctor discovered that "Twin A's" amniotic fluid was extremely low, which meant the sac was possibly ruptured. I could sense that he wanted to offer me hope, but instead he could only give me his medical opinion. Gravely he told me, "I do not think this baby will make it."

He also informed me that miscarrying "Twin A" would trigger premature labor for her sister. There was little to no hope that she would be able to make it so early in my pregnancy. Medically speaking, any real chance of survival was seven weeks away at twenty-four weeks. I was sent home on bed rest to maintain as much of the amniotic fluid as I could with the hope of preserving my babies.

At our eighteen-week appointment, we could no longer find a heartbeat for "Twin A." There was nothing the doctor could medically do to save "Twin B"—so I remained on bed rest. My husband and I did the only thing we could— we prayed!

My heart railed at God, "Why me?" I was tormented by thoughts of how easy it seemed to be for other people to get pregnant and carry their babies full-term. If I were God, I wouldn't have even allowed some of those people to conceive because from my misguided perspective, they were undeserving.

Realizing that my thoughts were poison, I determined to shift my focus. Instead of pitying myself and judging and envying others, I focused on remaining positive for our baby. I did everything I could to bond with her and assure her that it was all going to be okay.

With God, I made it to our twenty-four-week goal, and my doctors decided that it was best for me to remain on bed rest for the duration of my pregnancy. Soon after, I was admitted into the hospital, as my doctors were concerned that I would develop an infection from "Twin A," who was still inside me. I remained in the hospital until I delivered at thirty-three weeks.

As my liver enzymes began to elevate, I was scheduled for a Caesarean delivery. So on January 15, 2014, Dr. Martin Luther King's birthday, our precious "I Have a Dream Baby," Ava Marie Cleveland, was born at 4 lbs 8.5 oz. She was strong and able to breathe on her own! She remained in NICU another two weeks before we were able to bring her home.

Today, Ava is a super smart, hilarious, feisty sixteen-month-old! She is standing tall in the ninety-eighth percentile for her age range in height. My name is Nia—meaning "purpose"—and she is Ava, meaning "life"—her life helped me discover my purpose.

I am so blessed to have realized the manifestation of our dream. Along this journey, my faith was tested, shattered, and mended again. I like to compare it to the Japanese art form "Kintsugi," where broken ceramic pieces are mended using gold, making it stronger, more valuable, and beautiful than it was originally.

We never gave up on our dream of becoming parents. Everyone's situation is going to be different! Yours may require that you attempt some unconventional approaches. But if you endure—it can and will happen for you. All I can tell you is... Don't give up on your dream!

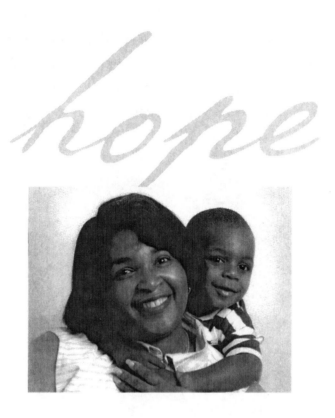

Hope In... The God Of Our Rest

*"You are my refuge and my shield; I have put
my hope in your word."*

Psalm 119:14

CYNTHIA-SYNDI PITTMAN

And On the 7th Day

otherhood for me began at four years old when I played helper to my mom with the first grandchild of our family. The extra work didn't bother me. From a young age, I'd been taught Bible stories about the creation of man. In my young mind, I was helping with God's creation. Although I was a very young aunt, it was plenty of preparation. My training continued as I took on the role of family babysitter, caretaker, and godmother.

I never questioned motherhood being a part of my future. But at the age of eighteen, I was diagnosed with fibroids and endometriosis. I was plagued with heavy menstrual cycles, debilitating pain, and severe anemia. The bleeding was so heavy that I always traveled with extra clothes in my car.

Like many other women, I just kept going and living. There was so much that I wanted to see and do that I didn't factor in the stress the fibroids placed on my body. I was determined that fibroids weren't going to slow me down or disrupt my life. Even though I tried to ignore the effects, others could see that there was something going on. I endured cycles of excessive weight gain and dramatic weight loss.

Being the youngest sibling and unmarried, my family frequently felt it was fair game to make my singleness and the fact that I didn't have children a topic of conversation. Holiday dinners and family gatherings became events where I learned how to dodge and hide from their inquisitive questioning of my plans to settle down and start a family.

Initially, I attempted to manage my fibroids through changing my diet. The right food choices helped me manage my weight and bloating. This went on well into my thirties. Becoming a mother was high on my priority list, but it was far from being my reality. I never shared my battle with fibroids and endometriosis with my family. I don't think I was ready to publicly deal with the possibility I might never have children. All of my siblings were contributing to the grandchildren pool. I didn't think my family could handle hearing the news.

My fibroid complications continued with excessive bleeding, becoming even heavier and more frequent. Then, one day, I began to have severe upper abdominal pains, which my doctors thought to be either the onset of a stomach ulcer or scar tissue moving into another area of my body.

One of my brothers had suddenly taken ill in Florida, and on my way home I experienced intense and violent pain that landed me in the emergency room. Sadly, my brother passed away, and in the week that followed, I was consumed with family matters and funeral arrangements. I played phone tag with my gynecologist, who was desperately trying to reach me for an immediate checkup.

I scheduled my appointment, and my doctor quietly explained to me that I didn't have an ulcer... I was actually pregnant! We were both astonished because I was less than two weeks pregnant. He was amazed that my blood work revealed positive test results earlier than usual. Immediately we began to plan a course of action for my care. There was no sugar coating the fact that the endometriosis and the fibroids put me squarely in the very high-risk pregnancy category.

Weakened by fibroids, my cervix was surgically stitched closed at the end of my first trimester. I was placed in the hospital on bed rest and monitored around the clock, as I had already started to present signs of pre-term labor. My doctor feared I would have a miscarriage, so I had to remain in a reclining position with my feet elevated higher than my head. He explained to me that because my body was so conditioned to heavy bleeding and passing heavy clots, that it was actually rejecting the baby. My body was preparing to cleanse itself and acted as if the baby was part of the thickened wall of my uterine lining.

Lying in that hospital bed with my feet up was tough. But I needed to keep as much pressure as possible off my cervix. Eating was a nightmare, but none of that mattered! It was all a small price to pay for my baby.

The remaining months of my pregnancy were the beginning of my personal transformation. I had lots of time to reflect as I remained in the hospital. As the days passed, I thought about certain events in my life, and I searched my heart. I'd had six previous miscarriages, and I was weighed down by guilt, shame, and loss. I repented and gave my life to the LORD, and I learned how to forgive myself and finally embraced new life—for me and the baby that was growing inside me.

Since I was confined to the hospital, I became creative about finding ways to bring the outside world into my little room. I couldn't go down to the main floor and attend chapel, so my hospital room became a prayer closet for everyone to find encouragement and strength.

My family was extremely supportive and moved game night to my hospital room, where I continued my reign as the UNO queen. I filled my room with the sounds of laughter and love. Swapping recipes, family stories, and offering encouragement to other women on the floor were some of the ways I was able to stay focused and strong during my hospital stay. I remained aware of my medical issues, but I was determined to trust God and believe that He would keep my baby—and me—in His hands.

Sometimes it seemed like the more I followed the doctors' orders, the worse things became. I had to endure negative report after negative report. It was the encouraging words of family and friends that helped me to hold it all together despite the intensity of the pressure.

During this time, I can honestly say I took life one moment at a time. I endured every injection, ultrasound, and visit to labor and delivery by reminding myself of God's faithfulness. Planning a baby shower was out of the question because we simply didn't know when I would go into real labor. All we could do was pray and wait!

On the day of delivery, the neonatal team was in place and ready. Just as I approached the finish line, we had one more scare. The umbilical cord had become entangled around my baby's neck. There was a quiet and stillness in the room that I will never forget. It's like we all forgot to breathe as everyone anxiously watched as the doctor worked to remove the cord. I was mentally, emotionally, and physically exhausted. My oxygen was artificially supplied...as in all other moments of distress, I did what I could...I prayed.

Suddenly, a screeching, tiny roar filled the room. My fierce fighting lion had made it through the valley of the shadow of the death, and he wanted the world to know that he was here! Doctors, nurses, and family all cheered! I looked at my doctor, whose eyes were filled with tears. He'd fought the battle with me every step of the way. He'd been there through all of my ups and downs. He'd stood by me as I endured the pain of losing six children before.

I lay there and marveled. I felt as if God had sent me a message. I was my parents' seventh child, my baby was born on my seventh attempt, and he was born on the seventh day of the month. It was a God wink!

Everyone stood by closely to make sure my little tiny gift was tucked neatly in his place—my arms. I named him Lawrence De'Jahn, a biblical and French name meaning King of John, in dedication to my late brother John.

Today, Lawrence is a twenty-one year-old college student working and chasing after God's heart. My fibroids continue to cause complications, but it's nothing that I can't manage.

Daily, I show my appreciation to God for trusting me to provide, nurture, and protect Lawrence on his passage to manhood. An endless "Thank you" is how I show my gratitude to God for allowing me the opportunity to witness and take part in such a miracle!

hope

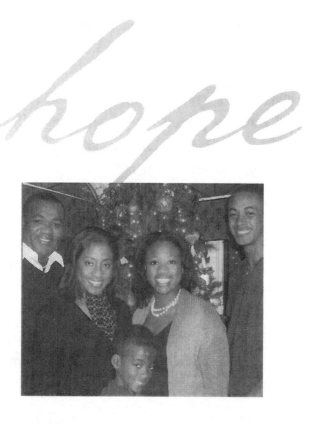

Hope In... The God Who Heals

*"But he was wounded for our transgressions,
he was bruised for our iniquities: the
chastisement of our peace was upon him; and
with his stripes we are healed."*

Isaiah 53:5 KJV

ROSILYN HOUSTON

By His Stripes, You Are Healed

In 2000, I was diagnosed with fibroids, six years after giving birth to my second child. I did not experience the typical symptoms or challenges commonly associated with fibroids. My doctor monitored their progression, as I had multiple fibroids scattered like "popcorn" spots throughout my uterus. I was not in pain, nor was I experiencing excessive bleeding. My major complaint was I had a belly the size of a woman near twenty weeks gestation.

In 2001, my fibroids continued to multiply but not increase in size. My doctor recommended a hysterectomy. As far as my husband, Ron, and I were concerned, we were past our child-bearing years. So we thought!

GESSIE J. THOMPSON *with*
COACH FELICIA T. SCOTT

A year later, we made the decision to proceed with the surgery; however, we then learned I was pregnant with our third child! It was designated as a high-risk pregnancy due to my age and the number of fibroids present in the uterus. Despite that, my pregnancy progressed with no complications, as my doctor was very careful to monitor me for excessive growth of the fibroids and to ensure they did not outpace the growth of our baby.

I successfully carried our son to full term with no complications at all during the pregnancy. However, a week before my due date, I began to experience pain on my right side. I mentioned this to my doctor, and he conducted all of the necessary tests and imaging, finding the baby to be healthy with no obstruction or reason for the pain. I was scheduled for delivery on September 26, 2002, by inducement and a natural delivery. During the labor hours, everything was calm and peaceful. The baby presented within six hours, and I was ready to give birth to our healthy baby boy!

Christian Devon Houston was introduced to the world at 2:32 p.m., and at 2:37 p.m., I bled to death after losing nine units of blood and flatlining on the delivery table. Normally, the uterus naturally retracts after giving birth, but after Christian was delivered, the doctor couldn't get mine to retract. It remained open, thus the bleeding was uncontrollable and rapid.

According to my husband, emotions plummeted from joy to pure terror while he watched in horror as blood flooded the birthing table and onto the floor. My doctor was caught completely off-guard and was both praying and recalling to memory everything he learned in medical school and from his twenty-plus years of experience delivering babies.

I was quickly whisked out of the birthing suite into the operating room, where they worked to resuscitate me. I came around and crashed twice in the operating room, so I'm told. My doctor wouldn't give up, and with God on his side, he was able to resuscitate me, keep my heart pumping, and stabilize me enough to perform the emergency hysterectomy necessary to stop the hemorrhaging.

Ron called every family member he could think of and asked them to pray. He didn't know if his last image of our lives together would be the horrific scene left behind in the delivery room. The doctors didn't have time to tell him what they were going to do nor come back to update him if I was dead or alive. He waited several hours while they performed an emergency hysterectomy to stop the bleeding. The procedure was extremely difficult and lengthy. By this time, I was 10 cm dilated, fully effaced, and my internal organs had shifted to accommodate the full-term pregnancy. No one would voluntarily perform a hysterectomy under these circumstances, but this was trauma and the only option to save my life.

Ron was relieved when the doctor finally got me stable enough to leave the operating room and provide him with the update that I was alive, but he didn't—and couldn't offer— any further consolation because I was critical.

Nothing could have prepared Ron for the sight he walked into when he was allowed to see me after recovery. I was in the Critical Care Unit fully intubated, receiving blood transfusions, and hooked up to a heart-pumping monitor. I was swollen beyond recognition, and I was not expected to make it if my vitals didn't hold steady through the night. I continued to struggle, swell, and my blood count was decreasing, which was quite perplexing because I was receiving continuous blood transfusions. It was later determined that I was still bleeding internally, but they did not know the source.

My doctor told my husband and family that I would undergo more testing to determine the site of the bleeding.

The tests revealed I was leaking in one of my ovaries and would need to go back to surgery. At this point, my doctor was not confident that my body was strong enough to withstand more trauma, and there was risk that I would flatline again. He told Ron that he would do all that he knew how, but I was deep in the woods.

My late mother, a praying woman, and all of my siblings and closest friends quickly came to the hospital. They gathered around my bed and began to call on the name of Jesus. We needed a miracle, and they believed God was not finished with me yet. They prayed the prayer of faith over me and released me into the hands of the doctor, knowing fully that Jesus Christ would be the chief physician in the operating room.

I was intubated and couldn't open my mouth, but my heart was full of faith, and I worshipped God in spirit and in truth. God sent an angel to my bedside. She was dressed in a white doctor's coat and whispered the Word of God in my ear—telling me who I was in Christ and that I shall live and not die. I could feel the presence of the Lord envelop me with the warmth of His radiant light, love, peace, and blessed assurance with each word she spoke. As nurses wheeled me out of my room and into the hallway, she escorted me, together with them, into the OR for my second surgery.

When I awakened, I saw her again with my chart outside my room while intubated in critical care. The nurses apologized to me because they questioned her and thought they may have insulted her. They said, "We didn't mean to offend your doctor. We just didn't recognize her. We've never seen her before." I was never billed for her services, nor did I ever see her again. Hallelujah!

God brought me through, and He brought me out. When fibroids threatened my very existence, He made a way of escape. I remained in the hospital in critical condition for ten more days. On day seven, I was just strong enough to be walked down to the maternity floor and was finally able to see my baby again and hold him for the very first time. He was beautiful and healthy. The Spirit of the Lord was upon him as well, and when I felt his little body next to mine, the Lord let me know that this child had great purpose and was sent to the world as a witness of God's faithfulness and the miracles that He would continue to perform on our behalf.

At twenty-three months, my son was diagnosed with leukemia. Today, Christian is twelve years old, healed, and thriving. I am healthy and living my life on purpose, walking in authority, and declaring the mighty works of the Lord, just as the angel proclaimed!

Selah. Or, as it's translated in the Bible, "Pause, and calmly think of that."

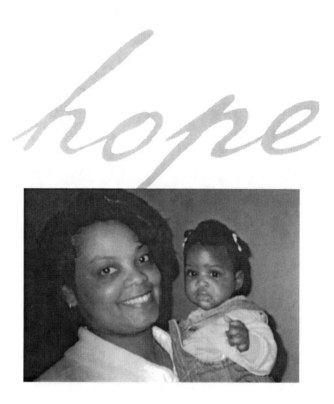

Hope In... The God Of Our Desires

*"Take delight in the Lord, and he will give
you the desires of your heart."*

Psalm 37:4

TRACEY
WASHINGTON-BAGLEY

Born From My Heart

I remember at a young age kneeling down at my bedside, praying to God, pleading to Him, to send me a little brother or sister. It took ten years, but God blessed me with a little curly-haired brother named Troy. Finally, I had a sibling of my very own; finally, I was a big sister! My life would change forever, and despite claims made by some adults that I would be jealous, I loved my newfound position in life as a mini-Mom.

I will never forget the call from my father to tell me about my new brother, who weighed in at 8 lbs. 12 oz. From that day forward, I realized the joy of sisterhood—in my opinion, a prerequisite for motherhood. After all, this baby I had prayed for was the center of my world. I learned to change his diaper, feed him on schedule, bathe him, take his temperature, teach him new things, and rock him to sleep. My early lesson in life was all about unconditional love!

I always imagined that someday I would get married and have children of my own. After all, I had hands-on experience with my favorite little person. After graduating from Ohio University, I married my freshman sweetheart. I recall asking him once when we first started dating if he wanted to have children, and he said he always thought about adopting a child. I found that to be impressive coming from a nineteen-year-old college freshman.

For years I suffered from severe cramps and heavy bleeding, often times leaving high school in a taxi because the pain was unbearable. I ignored my best friend's comments about dealing with the pain and preparing for a future career with an impeccable attendance record. Advil and Tylenol didn't exist at the time, and so the aspirin I swallowed was just an exercise of hope.

Eventually I was diagnosed with an infertility triad— fibroids, ovarian cysts and severe endometriosis, a disease that involves your ovaries when displaced tissue has no way to exit your body and becomes trapped and causes pain and sometimes fertility issues. Three major surgeries later and a cancer scare, a hysterosalpingogram (HSG), (an X-ray test that examines the uterus and fallopian tubes), my results revealed the worst news of my life—I wouldn't be able to conceive naturally.

Balancing my career as an award-winning TV producer, I held on to the possibility of In-Vitro fertilization, but after several failed, extremely expensive, cycles, including one implanted embryo that didn't survive, our cradle was looking quite empty.

I dreaded opening another baby shower invite. I recall telling my mother several times that it was so unfair that I couldn't give birth to a child of my own. I felt robbed of the ultimate experience of womanhood—motherhood. My mother, a New York City teacher of thirty years—responded, "Motherhood begins after a child is born, and when you adopt that child, he/she will be your very own!"

Little did I know that one day we would receive a call from the Family Options Adoption agency that a newborn baby girl in Long Branch, New Jersey, needed a loving family. The next day, I held a beautiful, bright-eyed, long-legged baby girl for hours that felt like minutes in a rocking chair in a nursery.

The possibility that she could become my very own daughter was indescribable!

Days later, after creating an instant nursery, my husband and I signed adoption papers, making Danielle Erin Bagley our very own bundle of joy. Looking back at my decision to become an adoptive mom and my former husband's desire to adopt, I realize that love has nothing to do with DNA and everything to do with GOD's plan. And when the question comes to mind, why me, my answer is, why not you? When Danielle was five, I told her that some babies are born from a mommy's tummy, and some are born from the heart. For nineteen years, I have been called Mom.

Today, Danielle is in college and loves to play the piano and dance. I learned from my journey to motherhood that when it comes to parenthood, God looks for people who truly love children and love them unconditionally—love them whether or not they come into your life by way of childbirth or adoption. He gives people a heart and the capacity to become adoptive parents; your love has to be beyond limits—it's a calling. If you want to be a parent, you can! Move out of God's way and let Him do His work. Unconditional love is real!

BEYOND INFERTILITY

Stories of women/families who suffered from non-fibroid-related infertility issues— stemming from complications such as endometriosis, an incompetent cervix, and more.

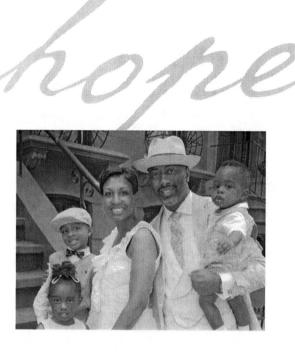

Hope In... The God Of Hope

*"Hope deferred makes the heart sick, but a
longing fulfilled is a tree of life."*

Proverbs 13:12

MICHAEL & ERIKA HUMPHREY

But We're Good People...

Our story began in 1999 at an after-work party in New York City. I met a beautiful girl at a Thursday night event. We exchanged phone numbers, and then Friday night we spoke on the phone for two hours straight. We had our first date that Saturday, and almost sixteen years later, we haven't been apart since!

Like many couples, we were excited about getting engaged and ultimately getting married in August of 2001. But we were on very different pages about when to start a family. If it were up to me, we would have started that process as soon as we got married—but Erika pushed back. She thought it was important for just the two of us to spend some time together before bringing kids into our lives. I was pressuring her hard, with various concerns about becoming older parents, as we got married at the tender ages of thirty-six and thirty-five, respectively.

Finally, sometime in late 2002, Erika and I reached a consensus about starting a family. We aggressively started on the journey of building our family, and pretty much the entirety of 2003 was spent trying to get pregnant on our own—unfortunately with no success. Initially, we felt that we were both physically fine, so I became frustrated quickly because we didn't conceive immediately. As part of the "fast food generation," I wanted to have everything I wanted "right here and right now."

Erika kept her cool and her patience but struggled internally knowing how badly I wanted to start a family. But at a certain point we had to take the pressure off ourselves and slow things down in order to bring our stress levels under control. The monthly arrival of Erika's cycle was constant confirmation that we were not yet pregnant.

In the meantime, family and friends all around us seemed to be getting pregnant and beginning their families. It's a difficult thing to see and experience! We were truly happy for our loved ones. Our smiles and hugs were real...but so was the heartbreak and devastation that came from the fact that we weren't experiencing that same joy.

In a blink, 2003 was over and the calendar rolled into 2004. We agreed to aggressively pursue a family again. And once again, we fell into a devastating pattern of monthly disappointment. I finally reached my limit and literally said, "Lord, I give up! I can't take this kind of constant shame and repetitive hurt and disappointment any more. I give up! How much bad have I done in my life that this is the extent of my punishment? You win, God! You win!" But I thank God that like the gospel favorite says, somebody prayed for me.

One night I attended a meeting of the Men's Ministry at my church, and I shared my testimony with them while I cried openly to a group of brothers. These men stopped the meeting, put their hands on me, and prayed for God to bless Erika and me with our hearts' desire for a family. The prayers of those brothers pulled me out of a very deep and dark place and let me know that I had to stay prayerful on this journey, honoring God with unwavering faith!

I'm grateful for my wife's prayerful and determined spirit. She realized that I was broken, and she masked her own hurt to protect me but kept praying and started the process of seeking a fertility specialist, figuring that one or both of us may have some physical issues preventing conception.

Due to my work and travel schedule, Erika first found and met with a fertility specialist without me. She prayed on it and chose a doctor and was later referred to the exact same doctor by her OB/GYN, whom we met much later. God was already at work.

A few weeks later, I was with her when she met with the specialist again. I was shocked when we arrived at the office and could barely get in the door due to the number of patients waiting to be seen. It was my first revelation that we were not alone in our trials and that fertility issues were common amongst all races, denominations, and socio-economic levels—infertility complications did not discriminate!

We had our consultation with the doctor, who inquired about how long we had been trying to conceive and told us about various options, including fertility drugs and IVF. She also put us on a fertility schedule, which included having both of us analyzed and tested for any unforeseen complications.

Erika was tested first and had a procedure called a hysterosalpingogram (HSG), which is a radiology procedure where a radiographic contrast-dye is injected into the uterine cavity through the vagina and cervix. The uterine cavity fills up with radiographic contrast-dye, and it allows doctors to see if the fallopian tubes are, in fact, open, or if there is any degree of blockage or closure.

As Erika was going through her procedure, I was also being tested and evaluated through sperm and semen testing. This involved an expert assessing a sperm sample for sperm counts, shape, movement, and various other criteria. This analysis was performed again a few weeks later to ensure and confirm the initial results, which were all positive.

Both Erika and I were given clean bills of health, and although we were both thrilled about the results, it also added to our frustration as to why we still had not been able to conceive. The fertility specialist suggested that before looking into In-Vitro Fertilization (IVF), we go through several cycles of the fertility drug Clomid. Clomid is a fertility pill that is taken to stimulate ovulation; it is used when there are no male fertility issues and no blockage of the fallopian tubes. We went through a total of three cycles of Clomid Treatment with no success.

Our next step was to attempt stronger fertility injections, which were difficult for me to even watch and even harder for me to administer to Erika myself. We attempted two cycles with these horrific injections, some of which Erika had to perform herself due to my work travel schedule. These injections were also unsuccessful.

Our final step before IVF was to attempt artificial insemination, also known as Intrauterine Insemination (IUI). We then attempted the IUI process, which is a procedure in which a semen sample is washed and analyzed and the best of that sample is deposited directly into the uterus and the sperm is distributed through a catheter. The sperm must swim into the fallopian tubes naturally and find an egg to fertilize. Prior to the IUI process, there is often a cleansing of the uterus. The IUI process also proved to be unsuccessful for us, and we were both devastated. I really felt that we had done everything that we could do, and we were both just overwhelmed, stressed, depressed, and somewhat hopeless about this process.

Meanwhile, more family and friends were calling with big announcements of their pregnancies. Even more heart-wrenching were the insensitive questions and comments from men and women alike. It's as if people didn't know any better than to ask questions that were none of their business. I marveled that people summoned up the audacity to say things like, "When are you all going to have some babies?" or "What's taking you all so long to have some babies?" or "Neither of you is getting any younger. When are you going to start working on a family?"

It's in those moments that I had to remind myself that I was a Christian to keep myself from getting physical or at the very least telling them to get away from my wife and me. Their actions were invasive, insensitive, and extremely cruel when questioning us about a very private matter!

I succumbed to the belief that children were simply not a part of God's plan for our lives, but Erika persevered. She pushed me to stay faithful and stay in the fight. She wanted us to strongly consider In-Vitro Fertilization as our last-ditch option. I was broken, but I was open to going the distance for my wife, so we began the IVF process.

In-Vitro Fertilization is the process of stimulating the ovaries to produce numerous eggs, extracting those eggs from the ovaries and placing them into a petri-dish along with sperm specimens, then allowing the eggs to be fertilized, and the fertilized eggs are incubated. Some of the resulting embryos are placed in a catheter and deposited into the uterus. In our case, approximately six embryos were extracted, three were used for our IVF process, and the others were frozen for later use in case this initial IVF cycle did not work.

We were counseled before starting the process that the standard medical practice was to utilize three embryos to increase the odds of a pregnancy. The hope is that in using/ inserting three embryos, the potential parents will have at least one cell take and grow into a baby that the mother could carry full-term. The doctor explained during our counseling session that with increasing the odds of a baby, by inserting three embryos, it also increased the chance of giving birth to "multiples," either twins or triplets. Wait a minute, did he just say there is a chance of us having triplets!? Oh my gosh, we NEVER gave that a thought! Three babies at once—No way! But, when we thought of how long this process and struggle had been, we quickly and easily made the decision to have the three embryos inserted.

We were so excited to even hear that there were fertilized eggs and embryos that were successfully harvested for our IVF process, but nothing can describe the sheer joy, gratefulness, and love that was expressed when the call came in that we were, in fact, pregnant with twins! We were just so happy, so relieved, so overjoyed that we were both in tears of joy and adulation. And the final stretch began, seeing to the responsibility of getting these gifts from God into the world.

Erika asked me, "Do you think you will feel some kind of way knowing that your kids were not conceived in a conventional manner?" My response was, "Yeah, I will feel some kind of way! I'll feel like a proud father because they are our miracles, and I know they are of God because He is the only real miracle worker. Our love is of God, this incredible medical science is of God, the people who prayed for us are of God, the hands of these doctors and nurses who got us to this point are all of God! So I will feel like a proud father whose ultimate prayers were answered two times over!"

And then, without warning, tragedy struck and totally tested our faith again!

Erika and I were thrilled about our blessings and couldn't wait to share the news with our families. Our parents and siblings were the only people who knew of our pregnancy, as we had been advised to keep that information to ourselves until we got through the first trimester.

Things were going along as well as can be expected, and
we were sprinting toward the end of the fearful grace period
of the first trimester! Erika and I were at home on a casual
and sleepy Saturday evening when I heard a bone-chilling,
blood-curdling wail come from my wife. It was like nothing
I had ever heard from her before as she screamed and wailed,
"MICHAEL, MICHAEL–I'VE LOST THEM! I'VE
LOST THEM–I LOST THE BABIES! I LOST THE
BABIES!" I raced upstairs as fast as possible, heart pounding
in anguish and fear, and opened the door to find Erika in
bed in a pool of blood. My heart sank, but my only concern
at that point was the safety of my wife. I had just never seen
that much blood before. I gathered her and helped her make
her way to the bathroom, sat her down and could see in her
eyes that she was in shock.

We called the fertility doctor and the OB/GYN, both of
whom said, "You're still in the game, but you need to get to
the emergency room immediately." We arrived at the hospital
on one of the Obstetrics team's busiest nights, and we waited
for some two hours to be seen.

Sitting in anguish and pain for several hours seems even
longer because you have a lot of time to think about all the
bad things you've done in your life. You start to remember

things and revisit old memories, and you question God. I asked God how He could take us through all of this and leave us now? How could God take us to such heights of joy and snatch it away from us now? I remember saying in my silent conversation and prayer with God, "But we are good people. We help others. We are honest, hardworking, nice people. We attend church, but we're also active, genuine, and faithful people, and we're working to build Your kingdom. Why this, Lord? Why us, Lord? Why now, Lord? Why would You hurt us like this? Punish me, Lord, but please don't punish my wife for my past ills."

When we were finally seen by the doctor, she asked what had occurred; once we explained, she said, "With the amount of blood that you have described, you have likely lost your babies." And at that point my faith kicked in, and all of my mother's teachings, all of my father's lessons, all of my grandparents' prayers over my life, all of my pastor's sermons all kicked in at once, and all I could think was, Is this the kind of Christian that you are going to be? No, because you are not a fair-weather believer. You know God will never leave you nor forsake you. Now let go and let God.

Just as the doctor began to perform her sonogram, I simply said, "Father, Your will be done! If the babies are gone, I trust in you that it was not our time, but You are still here with us, and we are going to trust and believe in You, so Your will be done." When that final prayer ended, the doctor said, "Wait a minute, I found a heartbeat!" My tears flowed freely, and all I could say was, "Oh, thank You, Lord, thank You, Lord, thank You, Lord!"

We got Erika home and got her into bed to rest, recuperate, and deal with the simultaneous feelings of joy of the survival of one twin and the loss of the other. And I did what any, grown, red-blooded American man would do in the midst of tragedy and chaos–I called my momma! I explained what had occurred and that Erika and I were really in some emotional trouble and that I needed her to help me nurse Erika back to health. And she replied like any mother would, "I'll be there as quickly as I can."

My mother and brother coordinated and secured a flight from North Carolina to New York on that Sunday—the very next day. My mother's arrival was right on time; she helped me and Erika pull ourselves together after experiencing such a traumatic event just the day before.

On Monday, Erika and I were scheduled to meet with her doctor to try to determine what had occurred and how to proceed. Once again, we explained the event from Saturday, including the blood loss and our experience in the emergency room. The doctor echoed the emergency room doctor's sentiments that with the amount of blood loss we likely lost the second baby. I prayed my same prayer, just saying, "Lord, thank You for sparing my baby's life. I know we were not meant to have them both, and I trust Your decision, and am so grateful that You will allow us to raise this one child as You would have us do. Thank You, Lord! Thank You, Lord, for this gift!"

As the doctor began her sonogram, she confirmed that she heard the one heartbeat, and then excitedly said, "Mrs. Humphrey, I've got a second heartbeat; both babies are still here! I've got two heartbeats; both of your babies are still here! Your twins are still here!" God had answered our prayers again. There was enough biblical significance in this miracle to last us a lifetime, as we had struggled with the perceived loss of both babies on Saturday, only to have one of them returned to us on day Sunday, and then on the "third » day of our ordeal, our God revealed the He was still on the throne, holding us up, as He performed another miracle in our lives!

We got through the duration of our pregnancy without too much drama, and on September 9, 2005, we welcomed

Michael Alan Humphrey Jr. at 4:00 p.m. and Melanie Imani Humphrey at 4:05 p.m. They arrived prematurely, at thirty-five weeks, and although Mikey left the hospital after only two days, Melanie remained in the hospital for a total of eight days until she reached the doctor's desired weight for her release.

Our lives have been blessed beyond belief by our gifts from God. We thank God for the miracle of our children. God blessed us with a boy and a girl, and our family was complete, so we thought...But God had other plans!

Three years after the twins were born through IVF, and following a relaxed, and much needed, vacation to the Caribbean, Erika informed me that we were pregnant again. On June 2, 2009, Christian Miles Humphrey was born, having been conceived without assistance. Erika was forty-three at the time, and I was a young forty-four!

Today, Melanie, Michael, and Christian are doing well! Melanie is into fashion and is a cheerleader and swimmer; her brothers, Michael and Christian, are both active in basketball. GOD IS TRULY GOOD!

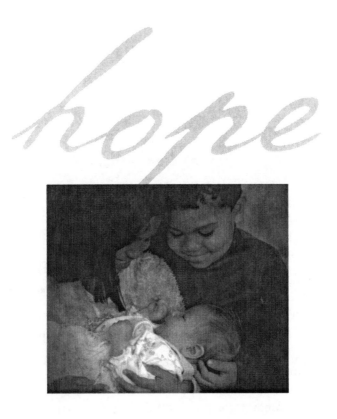

Hope In... The God Of Perfect Timing

"My times are in your hands;"

Proverbs 31:15

KASEY YULFO

Three's Company!

arcus and I were married in 1994. Two years later, we endured the pain of our first miscarriage. Though disappointing, the pregnancy was unplanned and unexpected, so we waited five years before we tried again. When it didn't happen in the first six months, I talked to my OB/GYN about infertility.

I started medication and monitoring my basal temperature. In 2002, we conceived again. We were elated, but our joy was short-lived. During our first sonogram, I knew something was wrong. I'd done my homework, and I knew what the fetus should look like at each stage of pregnancy. To my untrained eye, my baby didn't appear to be developing as it should be. My gut was sending me all kinds of signals, but I wanted my baby, so I ignored my instincts and allowed myself to believe the doctor's assurances that everything was fine.

Within a week, I began to miscarry. It was the most painful and traumatic experience of my life. We were devastated and waited another year before trying again. We tried everything that we could through the OB/GYN, including laparoscopy for mild endometriosis, sperm testing for Marcus, and lots of poking and prodding by various specialists to identify my problem.

The stress was too much, so we took two years off. We didn't use contraception, but we eliminated the pressure of doing anything specific to promote conception.

In 2006, we were referred to a fertility specialist. He took one look at my figure and diagnosed me with Polycystic Ovarian Syndrome (PCOS)—a hormonal disorder causing enlarged ovaries with small cysts on the outer edges that can result in failure to ovulate and weight gain. However, no cysts were ever found. Additionally, no medical reason for either of us to be infertile was ever identified. The doctor then began to outline the path that fertility treatments would take. After the exam, I told Marcus that I wanted us to take some time to decide how far we wanted to proceed before we committed to various treatment options. After thinking it over rationally, I decided that In Vitro Fertilization (IVF) was not an option that I wanted to pursue. Marcus agreed, and we decided that we would adopt if IVF became our only viable choice.

Our first fertility treatment was a round of Clomid to stimulate ovulation. Unfortunately, it was unsuccessful. Our doctor didn't want to try artificial insemination, so he presented us with two opportunities—adoption or IVF. Marcus and I looked at each other, then looked at the doctor and said, "Thank you, but we'll adopt."

Even before we were married, adoption was part of our future family plan. We wanted to have a biological child first, but after everything we'd been through, I had made peace with never experiencing childbirth.

By this time, I was over thirty-five and concerned about the complications of pregnancy at that age. I mourned the loss of never knowing a child born in the image of my husband or me, and at the same time I was excited to finally be moving on with our lives and our family. I had closure... I thought.

In the beginning of 2007, after much research, we began the process to adopt from foster care through a fantastic private agency. Our adoption experience, although nearly as stressful at times as fertility treatments and pregnancy, went smoothly. There were many hoops to jump through but no complications at all. We were truly blessed the way everything unfolded.

We received our foster license in May of 2007. Our intent was to only foster children that we would later adopt—we didn't want our home to become a revolving door of children. Over that summer, we reviewed many adoption profiles and submitted our portfolio for consideration in at least half a dozen cases. We were looking for a boy between the ages of three to five years old.

In September of 2007, we found him, but he came with an older sister. We were emotionally and mentally prepared for one child, but two? We didn't know if we could handle it. We reviewed their profile and fell totally and completely in love with both of them! We submitted our portfolio for consideration and waited.

Our agency informed us that there would be a court hearing and that a decision wouldn't be made until October. The month of October came and went with no news! The silence meant that the county had decided that our family wasn't the right fit. We were disappointed, but we continued to review more adoption profiles and submit our portfolio for more children. It helped to know that we were now open to the possibility of adopting two children at once. We could have our entire family in one shot, just as if we had twins.

We had to develop a tough skin, because it was disheartening to repeatedly experience the rejection of not being chosen as parents. We were excited when the agency asked us to consider taking in a newborn, but our hopes were dashed again when the birth mother decided not to put the child up for adoption.

In December, we received a call from our social worker. The county wanted to talk to us about the two children we had fallen in love with back in September. Our social worker informed us that things had not worked out with the other family that the county chose in October. We went to a meeting with several members of our county's Department of Social Services adoption team. Thankfully, our social worker was there every step of the way to support us through the process.

In the meeting, we were asked to explain why we felt we were the right choice for the children. We also learned more about them and their past history. There was total disclosure so that we could make an informed decision. There were several logistical hurdles to navigate; the county required that the children have separate bedrooms in our three-bedroom home.

Marcus and I took a few minutes to talk as a family, and we both felt that these children were meant to be ours. We would do whatever was required to bring them home. When the meeting was over, everyone was in agreement—we were about to be the happy parents of a son and daughter.

Our daughter, Elizabeth, was turning five, and our son, Joel, would be three years old. It was around the holidays, but we all felt it would be best to make the transition at the top of the New Year. The children had a foster mom who had cared for them for two years. We wanted them to enjoy their last Christmas with her.

We were nervous and excited to meet our children. On January 7, 2008, we met them face-to-face for the first time. It was exactly one year after we started the adoption process.

We continued to visit with the children over the next few weeks, and things were going very smoothly. We'd arranged to spend Martin Luther King, Jr., Day with the kids, but their foster mom had to cancel. We decided to take advantage of the extra time as a couple since we knew that our lives would change significantly once our new family members arrived. Specifically, we knew that intimate time as husband and wife would have to be navigated strategically.

While we were "having fun" at home, the kids' foster mom was continuing to help them prepare for the move. She asked them if they would like for us to be their parents. They responded with an enthusiastic, "Yes!" In my heart, I know that is the day that we became a family because it is the day that all three of our children chose us! Yes, I said three.

That was also the day that we conceived again. However, I would be halfway through my first trimester before I had any clue that I might be pregnant. Unlike my previous pregnancies, there was no morning sickness or other immediately obvious signs.

Elizabeth and Joel moved in on February 1. He turned four at the end of February, and Elizabeth had already celebrated her fifth birthday before Christmas. I laughed and joked with my friends about how great it felt to become a mom—without the dirty diapers and sleepless nights. They were independent and already knew the hygiene basics—brushing teeth, using the potty, taking a bath, etc.

As preschoolers, however, they seemed to have a never-ending supply of energy. In early March I began to notice that I was extremely fatigued. I'd been under some stress because red tape had prevented us from immediately adopting the kids, but I credited my exhaustion to first-time parenthood. I didn't think much of it until my husband's best friend commented on how tired I looked. It dawned on me that if he noticed, something else was going on!

In mid-March, I bought a pregnancy test—just in case! I'd never tested positive using one before, even with my two previous pregnancies. It was more of a whim than a belief that I could be pregnant. I didn't expect it to be positive. I took the test, and it left no room for doubt—I was pregnant.

My initial reaction was shock, which gave way to laughter. I'd buried the hope of being a biological mother. I truly believed that I would never get pregnant. We decided that if we had a boy, we would name him Isaac. We felt like Abraham and Sarah in the bible. We knew we'd been given a miracle, but I was in a state of disbelief and denial the first six months of my pregnancy. I couldn't embrace the gift I'd been given because fear gripped my heart. I didn't want to get my hopes up or become attached to a child that I could easily lose. I was so afraid we wouldn't survive another devastating loss.

But we were blessed, and my pregnancy was smooth sailing! There were no complications even though I was thirty-eight by the time I delivered. My labor, however, was complicated.

I had a natural birth. My contractions slowed at one point, and the baby's shoulders were so broad that she got stuck in the birth canal. Finally, she was delivered after fifteen hours— two hours of pushing—and immediately whisked away from me. Things happened so fast that I didn't understand what was going on. They never brought her over to lay her on my chest. All I could see was her feet as they were cleaning her. I couldn't hear that first cry I was listening for or anything before she was gone.

Shortly after, a doctor came in to explain what had gone wrong. She'd inhaled some meconium (a mixture of the baby's first fecal matter and amniotic fluid) during the birthing process, and the tar-like substance prevented one of her lungs from opening fully. Her lungs only had about 60% capacity. Even though the hospital had an extremely advanced NICU (one of our reasons for choosing this hospital), there was a chance that she would need the one treatment that they could not provide, and she would have to be transferred to another hospital.

We were told that our baby would need to spend at least one week in the NICU across town. It felt like an hour later when they finally brought her back in—at that time she was prepped and ready for transport in her isolette. God bless the nurse, who insisted the transporters stop by my room so I could see my daughter before she was moved. She was sedated to help keep her calm during transit. She was perfectly still, and her head was turned away from me so I couldn't even get a good look at her. They were there maybe five minutes and then headed to the other hospital.

Because I had just given birth, I couldn't be released to leave with her. The hospital tried to transfer me as a patient to the other hospital, but it was full. The next morning they released me at 10 a.m. By 11:00, I was literally standing by her side with my hands on her head and feet. I talked to her and sang. Before long, the NICU nurses realized that I had just delivered the day before and gave me a stool to sit next to her.

Even though I was finally able to touch Elena, it would be another two days before I could actually hold her in my arms. On the fifth day—her actual due date—she was able to come home. I knew that the older two children were meant to be ours, but Elena completed our family. I later found out that the adoption papers were filed with the court on the day that she was born. It wasn't a coincidence that the children chose us on the day Elena was conceived or that the adoption papers were filed on the day she was born. All three of my children are my miracle babies.

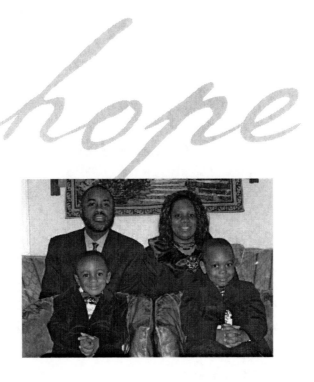

Hope In... The God Who Hears

*"But the angel said unto him, 'Fear not,
Zacharias: for thy prayer is heard; and thy
wife Elisabeth shall bear thee a son, and thou
shalt call his name John.'"*

Luke 1:13 KJV

SHARON ROBINSON

Thy Prayer is Heard

*L*et me begin by saying God is an awesome God. Webster's dictionary defines "mother" as a female parent who holds an authoritative or responsible position; to give birth to; to create; to watch over, nourish and protect. As I began my journey to motherhood, I knew from the beginning that I possessed the qualities described above.

My husband George and I had been happily married for twelve years. We had been blessed with so much and finally felt that it was time for us to expand our family. We had so much love to share, and we were ready to pour everything God had given us into a child of our own. But we didn't know that our faith would be challenged in so many ways.

In 1998, I was diagnosed with severe endometriosis, and the obstetrician/gynecologist informed me that I would never be able to conceive. Rather than crushing me, this news caused my faith in God to increase tremendously. The song "Whose Report Do You Believe?" became my heart's battle cry!

My husband and I refused to give up on our dream to have a baby. While seeking God for guidance and direction, we decided to get a second opinion. We found another obstetrician/gynecologist who performed a battery of tests, including one for lupus—and he found nothing wrong!

To God be the Glory! Science confirmed what we already knew!

We tried repeatedly, but month after month, nothing changed. Again, we consulted God and prayed for direction. I began to tell God, "Lord, you made my body. Do what you have to do to help prepare it for conception." Shortly thereafter, I conceived! We were ecstatic because the Lord had heard our prayers. We literally walked around in a bubble of excitement. But three months into the pregnancy, I miscarried. Although my heart was broken, I believed in God's goodness. I told myself, "I guess this isn't your time."

Despite believing that God would give us a child, I still had to deal with the frustration of waiting for Him to answer. Although I was down, I still took God at His word. I began to quote God's word back to Him. I remembered that the first doctor said that I would never get pregnant—God fulfilled His promise and I did, in fact, conceive.

Over the course of several years, I became pregnant three more times, and each time I endured the pain of a miscarriage—including twins in December 2001. I met with doctor after doctor, and none of them could identify the reason for the miscarriages.

Finally, I had to turn my face to the wall and travail in prayer before God. One Sunday morning, our assistant pastor, Bishop Clark, preached a message from Luke 1:13-47. He told the story of John the Baptist's mother, Elizabeth. She was a woman with a barren womb with no hope of ever becoming a mother. She was perceived as too old to even have a glimmer of hope of becoming pregnant. Despite these facts, the Lord opened her womb and she conceived a son.

I knew those words were for me! I sat on the edge of my seat and focused on the sermon as if my very life depended on it. In my heart, I heard the Lord speak to me. I was to read that passage of scripture every day in its entirety. I saturated my spirit with those scriptures, and with confidence I also embraced Luke 1:13—"For thy prayer is heard." God also laid it upon my heart to read I Samuel 1:28, the story of Hannah. I faithfully read those two passages of scriptures on a daily basis.

In January of 2002, I became pregnant once again. However, this time I was cautious and didn't allow myself to get too excited. Four months into the pregnancy, I started bleeding heavily and was rushed to the hospital. In the ER, they performed a sonogram—the baby's heartbeat was no longer there. The technician told me there was no sign of pregnancy—it was likely that I'd miscarried.

That was the final straw! I told my husband that I had reached my breaking point; the pain of carrying a child and losing it was becoming unbearable. I had done all that God had told me to do, and I could not understand why this was happening to me. I felt so empty and disappointed. I had lost all hope and reached the end of my rope. Little did I know that what I perceived to be my end was just the beginning for God.

A couple of days later, I started feeling sick and went to my doctor. He took a blood test and told me that my blood levels were very high and I urgently needed a D&C. Although I'd had several obstetricians over the years, I couldn't think of any doctors with whom I felt comfortable enough or trusted to perform the procedure.

So I told my doctor that I didn't have an obstetrician, and he recommended a good friend who was a top obstetrician at North Shore Hospital in Manhasset. I called her once I reached home and shared my medical history with her. Without an examination, she immediately told me that it sounded as if I had an "incompetent cervix"—a condition that occurs when weak cervical tissue causes or contributes to premature birth or the loss of an otherwise healthy pregnancy. Out of all the doctors I had seen over the years, she was the first to offer me any kind of explanation for all of the pain and loss my husband and I had endured. She also told me that because my blood levels were still very high, I had not miscarried!

Afraid to believe, I told her that I'd seen the sonogram with my own eyes—there was no heartbeat! She informed me that really didn't mean anything and that she would have to see me to determine what was really going on. God was in the plan.

After obtaining a copy of my records from the previous hospital, she called me back within the hour and told me to come to her office immediately. She assured me that I had not miscarried! My husband and I went in, she performed a sonogram exam, and praise God, there was a heartbeat!

My husband and I looked at each other in amazement. The obstetrician said to us, "This is your miracle baby!"

She immediately ran further tests, and her findings confirmed her initial diagnosis—I had an incompetent cervix. My diagnosis and medical history made my pregnancy high risk. Extra precautions and tests were taken to help ensure I would carry my baby full-term.

During the end of my second trimester, I was admitted into the hospital on bed rest. For four long months, I lay in a reclining position, feet above my head. I was virtually upside down! My incompetent cervix meant that my membranes were flowing downward (or my water was breaking). I had to trick gravity so my baby could survive. But I never gave up hope because beyond a shadow of a doubt, God had showed himself to be in control. I refused to lose hope or heart and determined to live life as normally as possible. I am a wedding planner by trade, so I used that time to work and yes, I planned a wedding while lying upside down on bed rest!

On August 9, 2002, our first son, George Cameron Robinson, was born. But God didn't stop there. I conceived again, and on May 22, 2004 our second blessing, Chase Jarrett Robinson, was born.

I am a witness to what prayer and faith in God's Word can do for you. When your back is against a wall, position yourself to that wall and pray. God's timing is often different from ours! But He is always on time! Always remember that you are a winner before the fight even begins!

BEYOND COMPLICATIONS

Stories of women who had no infertility issues but found themselves fighting for their babies due to complications that arose during pregnancy, post-delivery, or during the adoption process.

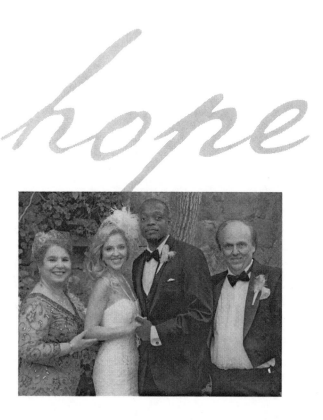

Hope In... The God of Impossibilities

"Jesus looked at them and said, 'With man this is impossible, but with God all things are possible.'"

Matthew 19:26

SUSAN DAWN COFFMAN

The Miracle Beyond Hope

*I*n 1980, our second daughter, Katherine "Katy" Mary-Elizabeth Coffman, was born in Enumclaw, Washington. She was one of two babies in the entire hospital. She seemed perfect in every way.

We brought her home from the hospital on the second day, and she proved to be such a good baby. She ate well, slept well, responded, and gave us so much joy. Then…it was a Thursday evening.

My husband, Bud, was at church teaching a Bible study, and I was home with my in-laws and our two-year-old daughter, Sandra. For some reason, I was abruptly moved to go check on Katy. I feel it was definitely God guiding me in that moment, because normally wouldn't have checked on her at that hour without a specific reason.

When I went into the bedroom to check on her, I noticed she was just lying quietly with her eyes open. Usually she would cry a bit when she first woke up, but she didn't this time. I picked her up in my arms and, with the other hand, reached over on top of the dresser to grab a new thermometer that my mother-in-law had given us that week. It was the kind you lay flat on the baby's forehead. I checked her temperature—it was 103.

I walked into the living room with Katy in my arms, but I still wasn't too alarmed. It was a new gadget of a thermometer, so I thought maybe I had to deduct some degrees or whatever to get an accurate reading. I asked my mother-in-law, "How do you read this thing?" She replied, "It's supposed to display the accurate temperature reading when the colors came on." Something just didn't make sense.

Katy was still just lying there being the perfect, sweet baby. I thought, if she was sick, she would be crying or something. Instead, she just lay in my arms, looking at me. I sat down on the couch, quickly reaching for the phone and called the doctor's office. I fully expected him to say,

"Everything is all right. That new gadget of a thermometer just doesn't read right." Instead, I heard major panic in his voice. He instructed me to immediately take her to the Children's Hospital in Seattle, about twenty minutes away.

I called the church, told them we had an emergency, and that I needed my husband to come home quickly. When he arrived, we loaded up the van with his parents, Sandra, and our precious Katy. It all felt odd.

We walked into the ER, and a doctor in a white coat approached us. He muttered a few things as he took Katy from my arms. Then he asked, "What's the problem?" I told him I thought she may have a fever of 103 and that she was thirteen days old.

He personally walked her back to a room and instructed us to stay in the waiting area. I couldn't understand the entire situation. I did mental checklists. I was young and healthy and so were my two daughters. A few minutes later, several doctors came out and took us to a room. When we walked in, Katy was laying still on a sheet wearing just a PJ top. They told us that they had done a spinal test and that she had spinal meningitis. I was told that I could carry her to her room where she would be admitted.

I felt the world move in slow motion, and I remember looking at the words that were on the little white PJ top she wore. In bright yellow lettering, it read "Take Me Home." Nothing else made sense, and I felt that's what I should do. To me, she was fine. I thought to myself, "Let's take her home and these crazy people can forget it!" But my body disobeyed my thoughts, and instead, I took her in my arms and followed them down a hall to somewhere.

A door opened, and I found myself in single isolation room. There they took her from me and laid her in a crib with metal bars. Nurses and doctors swarmed her crib, pushing me out of their inner circle. I just stood there, hoping for a glimpse of my baby through the sea of white uniforms that surrounded her.

After running more tests, her main doctor came to me and said, "Mrs. Coffman, she will not make it through the night. Go home! You are just making it hard on yourself." I felt the floor fall from underneath me. A nurse put her arm around me and whispered into my ear, "I'll be thinking of you." All my brain heard was, "I'll be praying for you."

I began to pray like all of heaven and earth depended on it. I never left the hospital while she was there. I stood around her bed, reading scriptures on healing promises, and I sang one song continuously—"There is Power In the Blood."

Over the next thirteen days, it seemed the entire infectious disease department came to view Katy. They put IVs in her head after the ones in her arms and feet blew. They continued to take spinal taps, which showed both viral and bacterial meningitis. She also developed a staph infection.

The doctors gave us no hope. I was only allowed to pump and feed her half ounces of fluid every eight to ten hours because of the swelling on her brain.

Then suddenly one night, Katy began to cry—a lot! She kicked her legs and screamed. She kicked so much that she rubbed her knees raw. My heart was broken.

While she was in the hospital, the doctors would not touch Katy. But there was one doctor who was different, a woman internist by the name of Dr. Brannon. She would stroke Katy's cheeks and smile and talk to her. One day, Dr. Brannon told me that the doctors were right about the results of Katy's test—one after another, all getting worse! Strangely, Katy's condition didn't match any of the symptoms associated with the test results.

According to the tests, Katy should have been totally limp or even dead. But Dr. Brannon saw her energy to cry and kick and rub her knees raw—to the point that they had to cover them with fleece padding—as some sort of great sign.

In the state of Washington where we lived, Mount Saint Helen's was blowing up! And a miracle was happening at the Seattle Children's Hospital. Our baby Katy was miraculously being healed, and on my birthday, May 22, 1980, we took our miracle baby home for the second time. What a great birthday gift; never better!

The doctors could not explain her recovery. One even warned me that we would be sorry in the long run because she would either be physically handicapped or never be able to walk or speak. I will never forget those words, because God blessed her to do everything the doctors said she would never be able to do!

The relief of being able to bring our baby home again was powerful, but just as wonderful as it was, fear had so gripped my heart. How had she contracted viral and bacterial meningitis and staph infection? Was it something I had done or not done? Would it happen again? Day and night I watched her breathe and lived with fear.

One morning I woke up and went into her two-and-a-half-year-old sister's room to get her out of her crib. She was standing up, so excited to tell me something. She said, "Mommy, Mommy, last night a man came into my room." I panicked and looked around, wondering what creep had come into our home. I asked her what he looked like. She answered and said, "He had a dress on." (I thought, "What?"). Then she said, "He pulled his dress up and showed me a hole in his stomach and told me to tell you that you didn't ever have to worry about Sissy again—she would be all right."

My mind went in a thousand directions: a man, a dress, a hole. The man was Jesus, the dress was a robe, and the hole in His stomach was where the soldiers had pierced His side on the cross. A man, a dress, a hole, that's how a toddler would describe the man she met that night in her room.

I believe with every bit of my being that Jesus appeared to our Sandy and spoke to me through her so I would hear and be amazed and know without a shadow of a doubt through the years it was truly God who had touched and healed Katy.

Jesus healed Katy 100%+, and He healed me of fear. The doctor's hard and negative words had brought me such fear and torment, but the simple words from God spoken to me through my two-and-a-half-year-old brought me peace to last a lifetime. As Katy grew up and was in situations that could have been very dangerous, I frequently remembered the words spoken that night and never doubted that God was truly with her, watching over her. He's been faithful to His promise.

Today, at age thirty-five, Katy—also known as spoken word minister "Oraia"—is walking and talking all over the world! She is a pastor and teacher and shares the hope of God with others. She has been a joy to us and to literally thousands of others. She's quite the gal—a true miracle! I could never, ever imagine life without her!

To this very day, I still have the little white pajama set that says, "Take Me Home" in my bedroom. We indeed took Katy home. Our family continues to share our testimony, praying and encouraging people to believe that miracles still happen, even today. Stop and recount your own blessings and the miracles that God's performed in your life. God is great— time and time again! Even when it doesn't look like it, God is in control. He hears our prayers, and I know He listens.

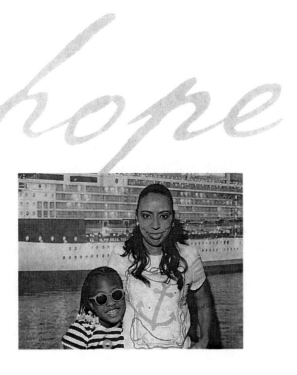

Hope In... The God Who Knows What's Best

*"And we know that in all things God works
for the good of those who love him, who have
been called according to his purpose."*

Romans 8:28

VEDA BROWN

Just Do It!

*I*n 1988, a struggling sportswear company introduced a new and memorable advertising campaign that soon catapulted the ailing business to the front of the pack. The company was called Nike. The unforgettable and now classic slogan was: *Just Do It*!

Decades later, that bold statement still inspires athletes and klutzes alike to work harder. Those three little words are a no-nonsense call-to-action, and for me, a personal mantra!

In 2004, my life took a surprising turn. I was a thirty-eight-year-old entrepreneur, and my business was bursting at the seams. I was "Single, Saved and Satisfied," with the t-shirt, the cap, and the bumper sticker to prove it. I had never married, didn't have any children, and was "okay."

I had been totally committed to Christ since the age of nineteen. Although I wanted to be married, I had no desire to become a mother. I didn't want to "slow my life down." I traveled frequently and loved it. I loved uninterrupted sleep and didn't want the responsibility that came with being a mother: a wife, yes; a mother, no.

I loved children—other people's children. I enjoyed taking them shopping and to Disney World, but I just didn't want any of my own.

But on a very cold day in December of 2004, I received a phone call from my sixteen-year-old nephew asking for a favor. His request was a far cry from the usual, "*Can I work for some money to buy gym shoes?*" Rather, it was: "They're coming to take my baby to place her in foster care. Can you help me?" My heart stopped for a minute. I took a deep breath and said, "When are they coming?" He said, "Tomorrow, on my birthday." Immediately, I hung up the phone and put on my proverbial 'Take Care of Business" hat. I happened to be wearing a Nike sweatshirt that said: *JUST DO IT.*

With my usual fierce determination, I called the Department of Human Services and was transferred and transferred until I was able to speak to someone who knew about the case. Then I was told, "Ms. Brown, it's too late; the parents knew about this two weeks ago, and the baby has already been placed with an agency. A foster mother is picking up the baby tomorrow."

I was also told that to have any chance of getting the child out of the foster care system, I'd have to appear in court in two days. The next day, baby Jasmine, who was just four months old at the time, was removed from the hospital where she had been admitted one month earlier and then turned over to the medical facility agency and her foster mother. Hours prior to her release, I held her, I prayed for her, and I cried.

Technically, Jasmine was my fourth cousin; her eighty-year-old great-great grandmother was my aunt, who raised me from birth and was living with me at the time. Allowing children to go into foster care just wasn't the norm in my family. When one of us goes through difficult times and situations, we all chip in to help. We always chipped in and helped each other and did what had to be done to keep our family out of the system.

Handing her over to the foster mother left a lump in my throat. At that point I had no choice; the fight was on. The slogan *Just Do It* became personal to me.

I resolved to do what was needed to help Jasmine's parents get her back. I became her unofficial advocate. I had no idea how hard it was going to be. Jasmine had been born premature and suffered a number of health issues that caused her to be in and out of the hospital for the first four months. The doctors could not figure out what was wrong with her and why she wasn't gaining weight. They assumed it was because her foster mother was mentally challenged and failing to feed her on schedule. Therefore, she was declared incapable of caring for Jasmine.

A court date was set, and I went but was told that I couldn't go into the courtroom with the biological mother. So, I wasn't given the opportunity to ask for temporary custody. For the next two-and-a-half years, I went to weekly visitations and monthly court hearings, fighting to get Jasmine out of the system. In the process, we found out that she had a missing chromosome that was passed down from her biological mother. This was the cause of her minimal weight gain and why she suffered from a low immune system, low calcium level, scoliosis, acid reflux, constipation, heart problems, asthma, and developmental delay.

I fought for Jasmine to be transferred to the best children's hospital in the country, which happened to be in my hometown. I tried with all my heart to prepare Jasmine's biological mother for motherhood so she could get her daughter back. I offered her parenting training in my home and argued on her behalf to make sure she received the services and assistance needed to regain custody of her child. I soon realized that the system had no intentions of giving Jasmine back to her mother because she was deemed unfit to take care of a child with serious health issues.

At that moment I went back and forth in my mind, trying to decide if I should adopt her, until one day, I took a nap and had a dream that Jasmine was *my* daughter. I woke up and realized I was wearing the *Just Do It* sweatshirt. I was more determined than ever to figure out what needed to be done!

I hired an attorney and fought with everything in me to get Jasmine, and the system fought back. Jasmine had become a valuable source of income to everyone involved, and no one wanted to lose that monthly income. During every obstacle, I always heard that small voice saying *Just Do It*, and I did. I just kept doing what needed to be done.

On my birthday, just one month before she turned three, I received full custody of Jasmine. Many nights over the past seven years, I have been awakened from my sleep due to Jasmine's acid reflux episodes or restlessness, but I'm really okay with it. I still don't understand why God "put the cart before the horse" and gave me a baby before He gave me a husband. But I've learned to accept that God is not programmed by our sense of order—or our timing. His way of doing things is not always "conventional."

There are a lot of responsibilities that come with being a good mother, but I continue to hear that small voice say *"Just Do It."* I do whatever needs to be done because I understand now that I really can "do all things through Jesus Christ who strengthens me" (Philippians 4:13). Many say that I have been a blessing to Jasmine, but Jasmine is a blessing to me! Together, we've been to the Bahamas, Jamaica, Alaska, and about ten different states.

When I received custody of Jasmine, she was on a feeding tube and couldn't run from point A to point B or get out of a chair without falling. She couldn't keep up with children her age. Her fine motor skills were extremely weak and her speech was impaired. Today, Jasmine is a determined, fun, loving little girl with a sparkling personality. She still makes about ten visits to the doctor every year, and each time we are encouraged by her growth and development.

Jasmine has surpassed all her doctors' expectations. They can't believe that she is the same child who first walked into their office seven years ago! She has taken lessons in swimming, kung fu, dance, gymnastics, unicycle, voice, piano, guitar, and drums. She's soaring and excelling—especially in language and singing.

With Jasmine, I've learned to appreciate the playground, play-dates, birthdays, Christmas, pizza, tacos, and movie nights. The "Me, Myself and I" attitude has been replaced with sometimes having a house full of children—and I love it! In the beginning, I thought I was doing Jasmine a favor by taking custody of her, but I soon realized that I needed her just as much as she needed me. I can't imagine my life without her.

I've learned to trust God on another level and to understand what it really means to totally accept the will of God for your life—even if it's not in your plan. I've learned to love and sacrifice to the point of no return.

At the end of the day, God wanted me to be a mother, and I believe that He orchestrated every moment of the process to make it happen. He allowed the obstacles and conflicts along the way to make me determined to fight for the child that was meant to be mine. Both Jasmine and I have a purpose in this world, and neither one of us could fulfill that purpose without the other. It makes me realize that sometimes God is waiting for us to *JUST DO IT!*

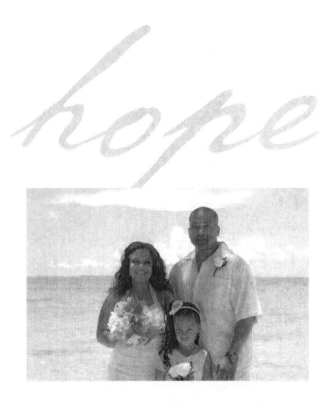

Hope In...The God Of a Better Plan

"Now to him who is able to do immeasurably more than all we ask or imagine, according to his power that is at work within us."

Ephesians 3:20

KAYLA TUCKER ADAMS

God's Plans for the Unexpected

I have always been the one who wanted to do everything "right." I graduated high school at the top of my class and went to college on a full academic scholarship. Four years later, I graduated with honors and one month later married my college sweetheart.

For me, marrying young didn't mean I wanted to start a family right away. In fact, having kids was never a big deal to me. My career was my focus. After all…I could have a child whenever I was ready. I couldn't have been more wrong. I soon learned that having a baby was truly a miraculous gift of life that could only be granted by our heavenly Father.

We were married nine years before I was finally ready to be a mother. In my usual "planning" style, I scheduled an appointment with my OB/GYN. We ran tests to ensure everything was in order, and I started taking prenatal vitamins six months before I wanted to conceive. Eventually, I began online fertility monitoring, and within two months, I was pregnant. Of course, I was expecting everything to go according to my master plan, but twelve weeks into my pregnancy, something happened: I started bleeding unexpectedly while I was at work.

I immediately went to see my doctor, and she informed me that I had placenta previa, which meant that my baby's placenta was covering the opening of my cervix, causing severe bleeding. As a result, I was put on bed rest for two weeks.

Two weeks later, I returned to work and resumed my normal routine. Two months later, while at work, I passed a large, clear glob after going to the ladies' room. Unsure of what it was, I called my doctor. I spoke to the receptionist, who put me on hold and then informed me that my doctor wanted me to go home on bed rest until our scheduled appointment on the following day.

The next day during my appointment, the doctor proceeded as if it were a regular examination and didn't even address my call from the previous day. Baffled, I asked her if she'd received the message I left with the receptionist.

She told me that she had been out of the office and hadn't received a message. Immediately, the doctor questioned the receptionist, and I soon discovered that the medical counsel I'd been given the day before was nothing more than the receptionist's uninformed opinion. Sadly, it was given at a critical point in my pregnancy, and those few hours made a significant difference in my baby's chances of survival. The doctor fired her on the spot!

I soon learned that I was actually in pre-term labor and would need to be hospitalized for the duration of my pregnancy. My doctor cautioned me that although I was in labor, the baby was "not viable"—she was not yet fully formed and would not live if she were born that day.

My doctor's office was on the first floor of the hospital building. In a whirlwind of activity, I was ushered into a wheelchair and pushed upstairs to the Antepartum Unit, where I was placed on complete bed rest. In a matter of moments, I lost my independence and was forced to rely on nurses to help me with my most basic self-care needs, such as bathing and using a bed pan.

Despite the best efforts of the doctors and staff, three-and-a-half weeks later, my water broke and I was taken from the Antepartum Unit to Labor and Delivery. I still remember the bone-chilling words of my OB/GYN. "Your baby is breeched, so you can't have her naturally. And at 23.5 weeks gestation, she is too small for us to give you a Cesarean because we would have to sever your uterus. What do you want to do?"

My heart and mind struggled to process her question. It seemed that she was giving me only one option—terminate my pregnancy—and for me, that was not an option at all. I told her, "Let's wait and see what God says about this!"

So we waited to see what would happen naturally. My doctor headed home, and less than an hour later, my daughter, Brooklyn, was born by natural childbirth. That day began an incredible walk of faith. She was born the night of October 11, 2006, feet first, in a critical state. Brooklyn came into this world at a whopping 465 grams—just over 1 pound—smaller than the average bottle of water. She had to be resuscitated immediately after she was born and was then rushed to the neonatal ICU.

At just 23.5 weeks, Brooklyn had just crossed the threshold into viability. If she had been born any earlier, the doctors would not have been able to help her at all. From the beginning, the doctors cautioned my husband and me that the odds were stacked against her. Our chances of taking her home alive were slim. At a time when my biggest dilemma should have been which shade of pink to paint the nursery, my main concern was making sure my daughter survived.

As you can imagine, from that moment, our lives were turned upside down. Confusion, sadness, guilt, depression—all the exact opposite of what we thought we would feel when we welcomed our first baby into the world. My husband and I spent a total of 149 long days in the Neonatal ICU. Those days were filled with few highs and many very lows.

Brooklyn spent five months in the NICU, with three of those months on a ventilator. She survived multiple blood transfusions, deadly infections, several cases of pneumonia, heart and eye surgery, pulmonary hypertension, feeding difficulties, and a host of tests, medications, and even experimental treatments to help her simply survive.

Once discharged from the hospital, Brooklyn required around-the-clock medical care. She had oxygen, an apnea monitor, a pulse oximeter, a daily regimen of six to eight medications, and required oxygen to breathe up until her first birthday.

My husband and I endured marital ups and downs during our difficult journey to parenthood. I later discovered that my husband often felt alone while we were going through all of this. Everyone was focused on the baby and me while he was suffering as well.

The stress of it all pulled him away. A year after Brooklyn was born, we separated, and eleven months later our divorce was finalized. Despite the dissolution of our marriage, we committed ourselves to being great co-parents. We decided to make every decision regarding our daughter together and to always put her needs above our differences.

Today, we are blessed to be able to say that Brooklyn is a healthy eight-year-old. She attends school, performs on grade level, plays the piano, and loves acting and modeling. She also takes Spanish and loves perusing eBay for Littlest Pet Shop figurines. She still faces some challenges as a result of being born prematurely, like vision problems, speech therapy, and chronic lung disease. But in Mama's eyes, she is perfect! The best thing that I hear at the end of a hectic day is my daughter sprinting to the door to greet me with her arms opened wide, saying, "Mama!"

Our faith is what got us through our journey. While in the NICU, we were told on three separate occasions that she was going to die—but here she is!

I am blessed to say that after being separated for four years, my husband and I remarried. We remain supportive and loving parents to our miracle baby. Every day that I spend with my family is a reminder that God still performs miracles!

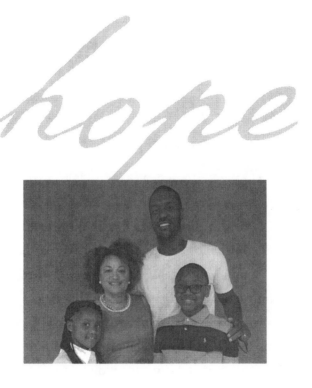

Hope In... The God Who Is Faithful

"Know therefore that the Lord your God is God; he is the faithful God, keeping his covenant of love to a thousand generations of those who love him and keep his commandments."

Deuteronomy 7:9

VANESSA M. GALBERTH

If He Did It Before, He Can Do It AGAIN!

Our son, Tyven, was fifteen months old when my husband, Todd, and I discovered that we were pregnant again! I was nervous because I had preterm contractions with my first son that began at twenty-two weeks. I was hospitalized for one week and released on medications that I had to take every three hours to stop the contractions. Despite taking the medication, I still ended up going to the hospital at least once a week for shots or IV fluids to stop my contractions. Throughout my pregnancy I was emotionally drained from the fear of going into labor prematurely. Tyven was born at thirty-six weeks and five days, and the thought of going through that again was overwhelming.

Once I had my first obstetrician appointment, my doctor reassured me that I only had a 15% chance of having any complications with this pregnancy. This put me at ease until at twenty weeks, when my water broke! I was laughing, right before my work shift ended, when, all of a sudden I felt a small gush in my underwear. I am a nurse and at the time I worked at the hospital in a mother-baby unit. I grabbed some nitrazine paper, which is used to detect amniotic fluid. The presence of amniotic fluid makes the paper turn blue. Well, my paper turned dark blue immediately. I was in denial and took another piece of the paper home with me. I said to myself, It's probably nothing. If it turns blue again when I check at home, I'll call the doctor.

Todd was not home, and I had to go to my mother's house to pick up our son. I checked again once I got to her house—needless to say, the paper turned blue. I called the doctor on-call and was instructed to go to labor and delivery. I drove myself back to the hospital and called Todd on the way there. I honestly can't remember the ride because I was so scared.

Once I arrived at the hospital, they checked me again. After a positive test, I was admitted, and my doctor came in to do an ultrasound. She looked at us and said, "I'm sorry." We were told that I hardly had any fluid surrounding my baby. She said that her lungs would not develop properly and that her limbs would be contracted if she even survived. The most likely scenario communicated was that I would go into labor within the next seventy-two hours.

We were given the option to induce labor, but since our baby was only twenty weeks old, she wasn't viable. We were also told that if at any point I showed any sign of infection, I would be induced because my life would be endangered. Aborting was not an option for us. We cried, prayed, and put it into God's hands.

I was to have an ultrasound first thing in the morning to get my fluid levels officially checked for exact measurements. However, within about two hours, the transporters came and got me for my next ultrasound. We paused; we were nervous because we figured God had not had enough time to work on our behalf.

While the technician was scanning during the ultrasound, Todd asked how much fluid I had, and unexpectedly she said that I had plenty of fluid! We were astonished! God had done yet another miracle for us and we were overjoyed! When my doctor made rounds the next morning, she said that she would like to see the fluid increase a little more. I was put on antibiotics and told to remain in the hospital until delivery. Instead, my amniotic sac resealed and I was released after one week...God came through for us again!

A few weeks later, I started to have contractions. I was again given medication to take around the clock to control my contractions. I was diabetic with my first pregnancy and again with my second. I was on oral medication and insulin to control my blood sugar. By this time, I was at thirty-four weeks, and, oddly, my blood sugar level normalized. In many cases at this stage in the pregnancy, the mother's insulin requirements increase.

At thirty-seven weeks and one day, our baby girl, Mya, was born. Ironically, they had to break my water to get her out! All the nurses were so amazed after she was born. They all just knew I would lose her. They said, "We read about the rare possibility of the amniotic sac resealing but have never actually seen it happen." She was perfect and her lungs were working—all the things the doctors did not expect of her.

Today, Todd and I celebrate both Tyven and Mya. Tyven is really shy and easygoing, but Mya is very driven and ambitious. God truly gave us two miracles...and we are immensely blessed to have both of our children!

BEYOND THE
EPIDEMIC

The story of one woman who has used her own battle with fibroids—and that of her mother's—to ignite a movement to raise awareness and funds for research to conquer the fibroids epidemic.

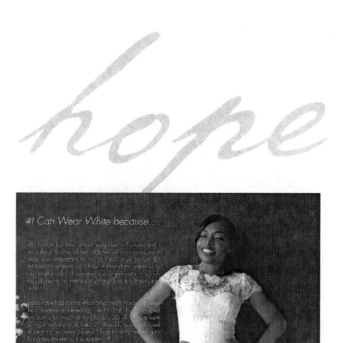

Hope In... The God of Our Vision

"Where there is no vision, the people perish:"

Proverbs 29:18 KJV

TANIKA GRAY VALBRUN

The White Dress Project

I'm not a mother yet, in the traditional sense of the word, but I sincerely believe my foundation, The White Dress Project (TWDP), has birthed a powerful story that is much greater than I am. In a relatively short space of time, TWDP has united a community of women and men who are dedicated to raise awareness about fibroids and build a movement to fight an epidemic that affects 70% of women in the US by age 50. I rejoice in knowing that TWDP will empower thousands of women to share their stories and heal from the physical and mental anguish of silently suffering with fibroids.

Creating TWDP has been my first journey to motherhood. In birthing and growing this organization, I've experienced a number of challenges and moments of joy that some would associate with being a mother: intense leadership, responsibility, and a burning drive to see what you birthed succeed. My desire to see TWDP grow into a healthy, long-lasting, robust organization fuels me daily to share my gifts and journey of advocacy to honor the life of my siblings who never had a chance to experience life. It also propels me more than ever to share the pain of my story and invite people to share their own experiences, while remaining optimistic in the journey to live a hope-filled life beyond fibroids.

Selflessness is a major part of motherhood, and I've delayed many personal desires to nurture and care for The White Dress Project. When someone asks me about TWDP, My Baby—or we reach a new goal—I smile from ear-to-ear. If someone doesn't see my vision or isn't speaking LIFE into TWDP, they better watch out! The White Dress Project isn't just another organization; for me it's my baby, and the story behind my need to birth her starts with my mother's own journey to motherhood.

Breast cancer and heart disease affect millions of women each year, but so do fibroids. In most cases, fibroid tumors are not cancerous, but they can seriously affect the lives of millions of women, plaguing them with a variety of reproductive problems and quite often interfering with the ability to conceive and carry a baby full-term.

When my mother was twenty-six years old, she became pregnant with twins and had a miscarriage due to fibroids. Devastated by the loss and unsure whether or not she would be able to have children, she chose to adopt my cousin, whom I affectionately call my sister. Deciding that the complications and symptoms that came along with fibroids were too much to bear, my mom chose to undergo a myomectomy. Happily, at the age of twenty-eight, she gave birth to me, her "Miracle Baby," on January 10, 1978—a special gift on the second anniversary of her mother's passing.

At the time, I don't think she was clear that I was her miracle baby because she thought she would have more children; she desired six, to be exact. Fast-forward a few years after I was born, and my mother conceived again—another set of twins—and sadly miscarried during her fifth month of pregnancy. After losing another set of twins and enduring various complications associated with fibroids—heavy bleeding, discomfort, and bloating—my mother realized I was her "Miracle Baby." She'd been pregnant three times and had lost four children; I was the only one to survive.

My father passed away when I was thirteen years old and it was truly a trying time for me. In hindsight I realize that I internalized a lot of the pain associated with grief. I never talked to anyone but instead held those painful moments in my body. I often think that the pain manifested itself in my body. At the age of seventeen, I started to experience symptoms of fibroids, but both my mother and I were in denial.

However, due to the heavy bleeding I endured monthly, I eventually decided it was time to see an OB/GYN. The doctor recommended that I have a D&C—a Dilation and Curettage—a brief surgical procedure in which the cervix is dilated and a special instrument is used to scrape the uterine lining and may help diagnose or treat growths such as fibroids. It didn't seem possible that a seventeen-year-old could have fibroids. But I did. My response was to simply deal with it.

Altering my life for one week out of each month became my life's norm. I created a checklist for when I had my period, and I never left home without the following items:

- Two pairs of underwear
- Two pads and a panty liner
- Girdle

In addition to my checklist, I HAD TO WEAR ALL DARK COLORS. I would NEVER WEAR WHITE.

Years of diligently following my checklist and wearing dark clothes for several days every month—not to mention four blood transfusions; a protruding and abnormally bloated belly; countless soiled bed sheets, underwear and mattresses coupled with embarrassing "leak through" moments (I always dreaded standing up when I had my period)—I knew something had to be done!

Fast forward to 2013. I was thirty-five and had been married eleven months, and I was still trying to enjoy the bliss of being a newlywed. My husband and I talked about starting a family, so I made an appointment with my OB/GYN to check the status of my fibroids. After a series of ultrasounds and MRI's, the doctor concluded that if I wanted to be a mother, I would need to consider the option of surrogacy.

To say that I was devastated when I heard the doctor's pronouncement would be a huge understatement! When the very role you have desired all your life is suddenly deemed impossible, it's unimaginable. I didn't know what to do. I was crushed. I questioned God and my purpose, because my opinion was, "If you're a woman, you're supposed to be a mother!"

I was overwhelmed by condemnation. I started to blame myself for not getting the surgery to remove my fibroids sooner. Emotionally I was in a bad place, but spiritually, I knew better and I knew that whatever was going to happen was supposed to happen. I was determined not to lose, and eventually I found a doctor who was willing to fight with me. We had a plan; I would take a DEPO shot to shrink my fibroids and then prepare for surgery.

But God had a different plan.

A month later, I started experiencing EXCRUCIATING PAIN. I believe the DEPO shot caused my fibroids to break apart, causing the pain. Within twenty-four hours, I was admitted to have emergency surgery to remove the fibroids. My surgeon removed twenty-seven fibroids from my uterus! I had never been told that I had that many fibroids; the maximum number I had been given previously was twelve— definitely not twenty-seven! My husband and I waited three months after my recovery period before trying to conceive and still…nothing.

During my recovery, I would research the symptoms I was experiencing, and I couldn't find sound, consistent information about what to expect or what to do post fibroid surgery. I did find a few blogs and heard tidbits of information here and there, but I didn't find concrete information about what I was experiencing.

I was desperate to be educated about fibroids and what I'd endured. I wanted to know the best strategy for recovery and what I needed to do to prepare myself as my husband and I tried to start a family. I knew that if I couldn't find helpful information then there were millions of other women like me who were desperate to learn everything they could about the effect of fibroids on their bodies and what the future held.

I searched for legislation on fibroids—laws about fibroid research, education, and awareness. I couldn't find anything. I was over it! I decided then and there that I was going to do something to raise the awareness. There needed to be a national discussion about fibroids.

As I thought about the organization that I wanted to create and the name, I knew that I wanted something that would grab people's attention. I'm a fashion junkie and thought, "I never get to wear white," because with fibroids my period was always unpredictable. Hence the name, The White Dress Project.

GESSIE J. THOMPSON *with*

COACH FELICIA T. SCOTT

The White Dress Project has allowed me to create a global campaign for the millions of women who have suffered like my mother and me. I wanted an organization where women would feel empowered to share their stories. I wanted to work with medical professionals and pharmaceutical companies to effect groundbreaking research and education for both physicians and women who suffer with fibroids. I longed to build a foundation that would honor the memory of the brothers and sisters I lost. Unfortunately, numerous women share the experiences my mother and I have endured, and my vision for The White Dress Project is for a fibroid-free future for women everywhere.

I'm not a mom yet in the traditional sense, but I have given birth to a beautiful gift! A gift that continues to give back, heal, and IMPACT women!

In 2014, my husband and I drafted legislation for "Fibroid Awareness Month" to be recognized in the state of Georgia, and later that year, a House of Representatives resolution declared July "Fibroid Awareness Month" in "The Peach State." Florida joined the cause in April of 2015, adopting the same resolution, and in March of 2015 the Georgia House of Representatives Resolution 612 for a "Study Committee on Fibroids Awareness and Education" was passed and adopted.

Now, even as I write these words, a "Fibroids Awareness Month" national resolution was introduced in the U.S. House of Representatives by Congressman David Scott (GA-13)! The work continues in Louisiana, the District of Columbia, Maryland, and across the country. These are all critical steps in honing my voice, sharing my gift, and my journey to motherhood!

Currently, my husband and I are exploring other options to become parents, but I realize that I may not have the directions yet for my journey to traditional motherhood. What I DO know is that I have begun my journey through the birth of The White Dress Project—a passion, an idea, and a movement destined to change the fibroids epidemic that impacts women, men, and families worldwide!

Hope Beyond Fibroids
Coaching Guide Excerpt
with Coach Felicia

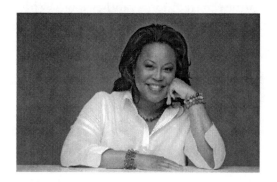

I believe in miracles. In fact, every day I witness one in the person of my niece, Nia Madison Thompson. Whenever I need a reminder that what seems impossible is possible—I look at her!

I believe that all of life is a miracle designed and crafted by the hand of God. But because we've figured out the science and processes behind some of His miracles, we have erroneously become convinced of our own control. We become falsely comforted by our sense of control, taking things for granted, and lose the wonder of life—until something breaks down!

In the case of the Thompsons - and the many families in this book - there was a definite break down! Life ignored their calendars and carefully scripted plans, and they were reminded of the limitations of their control.

I had a front row seat to the wrestling match between the Thompsons and the ravaging ramifications of infertility. There were times I was sure they would win, and there were some very dark moments when I wanted to change seats, because the carnage and the pain was almost unbearable to watch up close. I could fix nothing, so I turned to the one who could.

I don't have any biological children at this time, and am currently dealing with my own battle with fibroids. I am in my 40s, unmarried, and unsure of how God's plan will unfold to bring me the desires of my heart. I would love to be a mother one day.

This book reminds me of the options I have to that path and keeps hope blazing in my heart that if I endure my tests and challenges, a miracle is indeed possible for me too!

There are moments when tears of joy overwhelm me as I watch Nia grow and come into her own. When she puts her little warm hand in mine and pushes me off my agenda of productivity to make pretend pancakes in her little pink kitchen, I cannot help but worship the God who brought her here.

I knew her when she was the tears streaming down her father's face as he sat alone in his car waiting for his wife's D&C to remove the remains of a sibling she will never know. I knew her when she was the words uttered by her mother's pain-filled heart as she rocked on her knees asking for a miracle. I knew her when every holiday, for ten years, our family would link hands to pray and say, "Next year, there will be one more." And I remember when she was the awkward silence between us all because, for ten years, things remained the same. I knew her when she was nothing more than the unyielding tenacity of hope.

Infertility doesn't just strike couples—it impacts families! It is strange how something so very personal to a couple can quickly become everybody's business. Many never stop to think before asking couples and women questions about having babies. We, too, buy into the illusion that we get to decide when life begins.

I recall a Mother's Day brunch with family and friends a couple of years ago. There was a young couple with only one child, who was turning three years old. Suddenly someone asked the wife, "When are you having another one?" The wife and husband exchanged tension-filled glances. To me, the air around us had become hollow. But the other party seemed unaware of the boundaries her questions crossed. Their lack of response seemed to kick her into high gear, and then, suddenly, another family member joined in the barrage. "She's going to need a brother or sister soon. Are you worried about her not adjusting? Don't worry, she'll love them once they are here."

I cringed, because I read in their eyes what they weren't saying—more children wasn't part of the plan. As gently as I could, I steered the conversation in another direction. Our lovely brunch continued, but the wife was visibly shaken. While we sipped our chilled orange juice, she was left dealing with the aftermath of an emotional drive-by that had riddled her previous calm with bullets.

Some would say she should have ignored them, others would say she should have told them to mind their business... but the reality is that in moments such as these you do all you can and just get through it!

I was honored to be a life coach to Gessie (and Marc too, sometimes) on their journey. While I take no credit for the tremendous courage and dedication they displayed, I do know that I had a role to play. My expertise as a Certified Empowerment Coach™ gave me some tools to help them both through the process—and, when needed, to coach myself to a place where I could continue to be there for them.

The struggle to have children can be one that literally engulfs a life, a family, in a tsunami of emotions, medical procedures, stress and bills! It can consume every waking moment and become an obsession that leads to neglect and loss.

The purpose of this coaching guide is to provide tips and tools that will help you create balance in the eight key areas of life:

- Career

- Finances

- Personal Development

- Relationship

- Marriage

- Fun/Recreation

- Health

- Physical Environment

Each family featured in this book was asked a series of questions and their answers provided the framework for addressing the challenges of fibroids, infertility, and unexpected complications within the context of maintaining and designing a thriving life.

My mission in life is to help you Discover Your Worth, Do Your Work, and Define Your Wealth. Living well is hard work, but it is not impossible. Each day has a miracle for you if you dare to hope beyond your current circumstances.

Let's get going....

HOPE'S TENACITY

"Hope deferred makes the heart sick, but a
longing fulfilled is a tree of life."

Proverbs 13:12 NIV

This book was born out of one woman's need to give what she so desperately clung to in the darkest moments of her life... hope!

Hope is like many of the miracle babies in this book. It is fragile in the sense that you must guard it, protect it and be diligent over its care and your commitment to keeping it safe. Yet, despite its fragility, hope has a tenacity and resilience that can never be measured until it is tested in the crucible of challenge and difficulty.

Each and every family in this book faced a difficult decision at some point and time in their journey. On one hand, life presented a challenge, the facts and the known options. On the other hand, hope presented possibilities that remained unexplored. In that moment of decision, these families had to determine where they would place their faith.

One of the greatest dangers to any society, individual, or vision is the loss of hope. Hope sets the target for faith's aim. If hope is absent, then so is the possibility for something great and unexpected to happen. If hope lies sleeping, then real faith has yet to be born.

I am unsure of the reasons this book has found its way into your hands. Perhaps you are struggling with infertility or maybe you are supporting someone embroiled in that painful battle. Maybe you purchased it or it was gifted to you. However it is you found yourself here, one thing is key—you must have hope in your heart in order to move beyond where you are in a positive direction.

Sometimes we mistake outcomes for hope. It's critical to realize the difference between having hope and setting goals. Hope is the belief that it—whatever it is—will all end well, you are strong enough for whatever comes, and God will do what is best. No matter where you are in life's process, hope is imperative to your success and the unveiling of possibility.

If your heart is weary and broken, if infertility has stretched your finances to see-through thin, you are going to need hope to stay in the fight until you win. I always remind my clients that inspiration without action is nothing more than a good feeling. Transformation is only experienced when inspiration meets action.

Today, I encourage you to take your hope beyond where it has been by taking action.

Hope To It:

Take 15-30 minutes alone and answer the following questions:

1. What does hope mean to you?

2. What are the greatest threats to your hope?

3. Why do you have reason to hope?

4. Who can help you protect your hope?

5. How can you help others protect their hope?

**Download the full FREE
HOPE Beyond Fibroids Coaching Guide NOW
at GessieThompson.com/HopeCoaching**

AFTERWORD

*T*he sojourn to motherhood is unique to each woman, carrying with it awe and mystery. For most, it is a time of joy and celebration. For others, it is a journey that is filled with heartache, tears, and tremendous loss. For all, it is a time of immense anticipation and change. While on the surface it may appear that procreation is an easy task, the inner struggle that so many go through is just that—it is INNER. When the invitations to baby showers pile up and bright-eyed children are running everywhere, it is almost taboo to break that joy with your personal struggle. However, as the stories of these brave women in HOPE BEYOND FIBROIDS illustrate, victory awaits at the end for those who hope and pray.

These personal narratives illustrate the incredible medical challenges that couples, but most specifically women, face in the seemingly natural process of human reproduction. Amongst the various etiologies for infertility, fibroids are the biggest culprit. Fibroids are essentially parasites that live in our bodies, unfairly favoring African American and Hispanic women. Awareness, early detection, and cure are paramount to reproductive success in women with fibroids. As you read in these narratives, endometriosis, scar tissue, and blocked tubes are just some of the other problems that these brave women have encountered. Many doctor's visits, bills, medical procedures, and surgeries later, they have conquered them with perseverance.

No matter the cause of infertility, we live in a time where medical advances are so tremendous that what was once deemed impossible can now be made a reality. Procedures such as intrauterine insemination and in vitro fertilization have revolutionized (in)fertility with more and more couples seeking them. The field of reproductive endocrinology has fulfilled many a dream of being called mom and dad.

Despite the aid of medical technology, the stories of these women tell of the supreme God who is at work in the most intimate details of our lives. Human conception and birth is not a perfect science, despite medicine trying to forge it so. The answers are not packaged in ways that we may expect… but they are simply perfect at the end. Trusting and obeying our sovereign God is what we are called to do, just leave the rest up to Him.

As women, our ability to bear children is a high calling and gift. No matter our background, it is a yearning that tugs at our souls. Let us encourage each other with our experiences, may they speak to our very core and lift us up. I pray that each of us, like the families in *HOPE BEYOND FIBROIDS: Stories of Miracle Babies & the Journey to Motherhood*, is victorious at the end, filled with glorious peace and satisfaction.

Dr. Cheruba Prabakar, M.D.
OB/GYN & Minimally
Trained Surgeon
(DrCheruba.com)

Fibroids FAQ
with Dr. Cheruba Prabakar

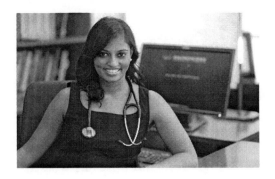

1. What are fibroids?

Fibroids are balls of smooth muscle tissue that grow in
the uterus. They are usually benign, but rarely can be cancerous. Fibroids can grow on the surface of the uterus, within
the wall of the uterus, or inside the uterine cavity.

2. *Who gets fibroids?*

Fibroids mostly affect women in their reproductive years. However, they can continue to cause symptoms until a woman reaches menopause. While fibroids occur in women of all races and ethnicities, for reasons that remain unclear, black women are disproportionately affected by them. There is ongoing research in this particular area and we hope we will reach a better understanding soon.

3. *How common are fibroids?*

Fibroids are more common than you may think. According to the U.S. National Institutes of Health (NIH), 20-25% of women of reproductive age have fibroids. By the age of fifty, up to 60% Asian and Hispanic women, 70% of white women and up to 80% of African American women will have fibroids. Uterine fibroids are most common in women who are in their 40s and early 50s, although some women may develop fibroids at a younger age.

4. How will I know if I have fibroids?

Fibroids typically cause heavy menstrual bleeding and this is what leads a woman to seek help. They can also cause pelvic pressure and pain. Fibroids can grow to large sizes and even make a woman appear pregnant. Depending on the size and location, sometimes fibroids may not cause any noticeable symptoms.

5. How are fibroids diagnosed?

Fibroids can be diagnosed most easily with a sonogram. Small fibroids that are within the uterine cavity can be better seen with a sono hysterogram—a sonogram done while infusing some water into the uterine cavity. The liquid distends the uterus and helps visualize small fibroids. Before undergoing surgery for fibroids, a Magnetic Resonance Image (MRI) is also frequently performed in order to visualize them better.

6. *If I have fibroids, do I have to have them removed?*

If you are diagnosed with fibroids, whether you want to remove them, or not, depends on several factors. The location of the fibroid(s) and the symptoms they cause are the most important factors in determining whether the fibroid(s) should be removed. Fibroids within the uterine cavity can cause heavy bleeding and infertility and are best removed. Fibroids located on the surface of the uterus or within the wall can cause pain and pressure. If the fibroids are entirely asymptomatic, there is no need to remove them.

7. *What kinds of treatments exist for fibroids?*

Fibroids can be treated medically and surgically. Medical treatment such as oral contraceptive pills, and other hormonal pills and injections can all help minimize symptoms such as heavy bleeding and pressure caused by fibroids. Uterine Artery Embolization (UAE) is also an option, where the blood supply to the fibroids are cut off via a catheter inserted in the groin. If medical and conservative surgical managements fail or if the fibroid is too large, surgery can be performed. For women desiring to preserve their fertility, a myomectomy or removal of fibroids can be performed, and for those who have completed child bearing, a hysterectomy is recommended.. These surgeries can be done via a traditional open technique or a minimally invasive approach. When feasible, a laparoscopic or robotic approach provides a better cosmetic outcome, faster recovery, and less scar tissue.

8. How do fibroids affect my ability to have children?

Location is key! Whether fibroids affect your fertility or not depends on where in the uterus they are located. Fibroids within the uterine cavity can interfere with implantation, preventing the development of a normal pregnancy. These fibroids can also result in early miscarriage. Fibroids that are located within the wall of the uterus or on the surface do not interfere with your ability to get pregnant but may affect your ability to carry the baby to term.

9. How do fibroids affect my pregnancy once I successfully conceive?

Fibroids that are located within the uterine cavity can result in early miscarriage as they interfere with the normal development of the fertilized embryo. Some fibroids also grow during pregnancy. Depending on the size of the fibroid, your doctor may advise you to remove them prior to pregnancy. Fibroids that are within the wall of the uterus can grow to large sizes and press on the growing fetus. This may interfere with normal fetal growth and development. As the available blood supply goes toward the growing fetus, some fibroids lose their blood supply causing the fibroid to degenerate or die. When this happens there is inflammation in the area and this process can cause severe pain to the mother. The pain can be so severe that hospitalization may be required for pain management. This process can also result in contractions and preterm labor.

10. Can fibroids be cancerous?

Fibroids are mostly benign. Less than 1% of them may be cancerous, although this is extremely rare. Unfortunately there is no way of knowing with certainty if a fibroid is cancerous prior to removing it. Gynecologists have developed new ways of removing fibroids without spilling or scattering pieces of it throughout the abdomen, in the rare event that it may be cancerous.

11. What is the earliest age women should inquire/get checked out for early fibroid detection?

There is no set age at which women should be screened for fibroids. However, women should pay close attention to abnormal bleeding patterns early on. If periods are very heavy with a lot of blood clots, this should prompt a visit to the gynecologist. Fibroids are a common culprit when it comes to heavy and abnormal bleeding in young women. They can be easily diagnosed with a sonogram, and treatment can be initiated quickly. Pelvic pain or pressure are symptoms that should prompt one to get screened for fibroids.

12. *What can women do to prevent the development or return of fibroids?*

Unfortunately there is nothing women can do at this time to prevent the development or return of fibroids. Paying close attention to symptoms can lead to early diagnosis and treatment. This in turn leads to a better quality of life. Once the diagnosis of fibroids is made it is important to monitor their growth. If the fibroids get too large surgery may be necessary. If fibroids are removed in preparation for pregnancy it is important to plan a pregnancy relatively soon after, as the fibroids may return.

Glossary of Terms

1. **40 Weeks / Full-term Pregnancy:** *To help more babies be born healthy, the American College of Obstetricians and Gynecologists (ACOG) and the Society for Maternal-Fetal Medicine (SMFM) recently changed the way they define births that happen after 37 weeks of pregnancy. Pregnancy usually lasts about 40 weeks (280 days) from the first day of your last menstrual period (also called LMP) to your due date. Your due date is the date that your provider thinks you will have your baby. ACOG and SMFM now define a full-term pregnancy as a pregnancy that lasts between 39 weeks, 0 days and 40 weeks 6 days. Babies born full term have the best chance of being healthy, compared with babies born earlier or later.*

2. **Amniotic Fluid:** *Amniotic fluid is a clear, slightly yellowish liquid that surrounds the unborn baby (fetus) during pregnancy. It is contained in the amniotic sac.*

HOPE BEYOND FIBROIDS

3. **Anemic / Anemia:** *Anemia is a condition in which you don't have enough healthy red blood cells to carry adequate oxygen to your tissues. Having anemia may make you feel tired and weak.*

4. **Anesthesia:** *General anesthesia makes you both unconscious and unable to feel pain during medical procedures. General anesthesia is commonly produced by a combination of intravenous drugs and inhaled gasses (anesthetics).*

5. **Antepartum Unit:** *Antepartum means "before birth." You may be admitted to the Antepartum Unit for Special Care Pregnancies if your doctor decides that it is necessary to monitor you or your baby's health status, to identify risk factors to treat complications, or to increase surveillance to prevent further problems. Your stay on the unit for Special Care Pregnancies may be continuous until delivery or you may be discharged and asked to return intermittently or frequently depending on the circumstances.*

6. **Caesarean Delivery / C-Section:** *Cesarean delivery— also known as a C-section—is a surgical procedure used to deliver a baby through an incision in the mother's abdomen and a second incision in the mother's uterus. A C-section might be planned ahead of time if you develop pregnancy*

complications or you've had a previous C-section and aren't considering vaginal birth after cesarean (VBAC). Often, however, the need for a first-time C-section doesn't become obvious until labor is under way.

7. **Capsule Endoscopy:** *Capsule Endoscopy lets your doctor examine the lining of the middle part of your gastrointestinal tract, which includes the three portions of the small intestine (duodenum, jejunum, ileum). Your doctor will give you a pill sized video camera for you to swallow. This camera has its own light source and takes pictures of your small intestine as it passes through. These pictures are sent to a small recording device you have to wear on your body.*

8. **Catheter:** *A flexible plastic tube (a catheter) inserted into the bladder that remains ("dwells") there to provide continuous urinary drainage. This meaning is for "foley catheter." Otherwise, a catheter is not specific for urine.*

9. **Clomid:** *trademark for a nonsteroidal fertility drug (clomiphene citrate). This medication is often the first-line therapy for women who don't ovulate and thus cannot achieve pregnancy.*

10. **Colonoscopy:** *A colonoscopy is a test that allows your doctor to look at the inner lining of your large intestine (rectum and colon). He or she uses a thin, flexible tube called a colonoscope to look at the colon. A colonoscopy helps find ulcers, colon polyps, tumors, and areas of inflammation or bleeding.*

11. **CT-Scan / CAT Scan:** *A computerized tomography (CT) scan combines a series of X-ray images taken from different angles and uses computer processing to create cross-sectional images, or slices, of the bones, blood vessels and soft tissues inside your body. CT scan images provide more detailed information than plain X-rays do. A CT scan has many uses, but is particularly well-suited to quickly examine people who may have internal injuries from car accidents or other types of trauma. A CT scan can be used to visualize nearly all parts of the body and is used to diagnose disease or injury as well as to plan medical, surgical or radiation treatment.*

12. **Dilation & Curretage (D&C):** *Dilation and curettage (D&C) is a procedure to remove tissue from inside your uterus. Doctors perform dilation and curettage to diagnose and treat certain uterine conditions—such as heavy bleeding—or*

to clear the uterine lining after a miscarriage or abortion.

13. **Dilaudid:** *A narcotic pain reliever used to treat moderate to severe pain.*

14. **Embryo:** *An organism in the early stages of growth and differentiation, from fertilization to the beginning of the third month of pregnancy (in humans). After that point in time, an embryo is called a fetus.*

15. **Endometriosis:** *Endometriosis is an often painful disorder in which tissue that normally lines the inside of your uterus—the endometrium—grows outside your uterus (endometrial implant). Endometriosis most commonly involves your ovaries, bowel or the tissue lining your pelvis. Rarely, endometrial tissue may spread beyond your pelvic region.*

16. **Endometrium:** *The mucous membrane that lines the inside of the uterus (womb). The endometrium changes throughout the menstrual cycle. It becomes thick and rich with blood vessels to prepare for pregnancy. If the woman does not get pregnant, part of the endometrium is shed, causing menstrual bleeding (period).*

17. **Endoscopy:** *A nonsurgical procedure used to examine a person's digestive tract. Using an endoscope, a flexible tube with a light and camera attached to it, your doctor can view pictures of your digestive tract on a color TV monitor.*

18. **Enteroscopy:** *A gastrointestinal procedure that uses of a flexible instrument (a "scope") to examine the small intestine, a very long hollow tube located between the stomach and colon (large intestine) and made up of the duodenum, jejunum, and ileum.*

19. **Fallopian Tubes:** *A tube that transport the egg from the ovary to the uterus (the womb). Each woman has two. In the diagram, the Fallopian tubes are not labeled but are well shown running between the uterus and ovaries.*

20. **Fibroid / Fibroid *Tumor* / *Uterine Fibroids:* Uterine fibroids** *are noncancerous growths of the uterus that often appear during childbearing years. Also called leiomyomas (lie-o-my-O-muhs) or myomas, uterine fibroids aren't associated with an increased risk of uterine cancer and almost never develop into cancer.*

21. **Flatline:** *to register on an electronic monitor as having no brain waves or heartbeat; to die; to be in the state of no progress or advancement*

22. **Gastrointestinal Bleeding (GI Bleeding):** *A symptom of a disorder in your digestive tract. The blood often appears in stool or vomit but isn't always visible. The level of bleeding can range from mild to severe and life-threatening. Finding the cause of GI bleeding can be difficult. Sophisticated imaging technology can usually locate the problem, and minimally invasive procedures often can fix it.*

23. **Gestational Diabetes:** *Gestational diabetes develops during pregnancy (gestation). Like other types of diabetes, gestational diabetes affects how your cells use sugar (glucose). Gestational diabetes causes high blood sugar that can affect your pregnancy and your baby's health. Expectant moms can help control gestational diabetes by eating healthy foods, exercising and, if necessary, taking medication.. In gestational diabetes, blood sugar usually returns to normal soon after delivery, but the risk of type 2 diabetes remains high.*

24. **Gynecologist (GYN):** *A gynecologist is a physician who has a successfully completed specialized education and training in the health of the female reproductive system, including*

the diagnosis and treatment of disorders and diseases. Typically, the education and training for both fields occurs concurrently. An obstetrician/gynecologist is a physician specialist who provides medical and surgical care to women and has particular expertise in pregnancy, childbirth, and disorders of the reproductive system. This includes preventative care, prenatal care, detection of sexually transmitted diseases, Pap test screening, family planning, etc.

25. **Hematologist:** *A physician specializing in hematology. Hematology is a branch of medicine concerning the study of blood, the blood-forming organs, and blood diseases. The word "heme" comes from the Greek for blood. Hematology is practiced by specialists in the field who deal with the diagnosis, treatment and overall management of people with blood disorders ranging from anemia to blood cancer.*

26. **Hemoglobin:** *The oxygen-carrying pigment and predominant protein in the red blood cells.*

27. **Hysterectomy:** *A hysterectomy is an operation to remove a woman's uterus. A woman may have a hysterectomy for different reasons, including: uterine fibroids, endometriosis, abnormal vaginal bleeding, chronic pelvic pain, Adenomyosis, or cancer of the female pelvic organs.*

28. **Hysterosalpingogram (HSG):** *An X-ray test that looks at the inside of the uterus and fallopian tubes in order to diagnose any abnormalities of the uterine cavity or to check for blockage of the tubes. It is an important step in an infertility workup.*

29. **Hysteroscopic Myomectomy:** *A myomectomy is a surgery to remove fibroids without taking out the healthy tissue of the uterus. It is best for women who wish to have children after treatment for their fibroids or who wish to keep their uterus for other reasons. You can become pregnant after myomectomy. This procedure is considered standard of care for removing fibroids and preserving the uterus. Myomectomy has traditionally been performed through a large abdominal incision, however advances in technology have provided less invasive alternatives such as hysteroscopic and laparoscopic myomectomies. While this procedure is more invasive and time consuming for the surgeon, it affords patients the opportunity to remain fertile. A hysteroscopic myomectomy removes fibroids through the vagina.*

30. **Hysterosonogram:** An ultrasound that is performed after first instilling water into the uterine cavity. This type of ultrasound enables one to identify small fibroids or polyps in the uterine cavity.

31. **In Vitro Fertilization:** *In vitro fertilization (IVF) is a complex series of procedures used to treat fertility or genetic problems and assist with the conception of a child. During IVF, mature eggs are collected (retrieved) from your ovaries and fertilized by sperm in a lab. Then the fertilized egg (embryo) or eggs are implanted in your uterus. One cycle of IVF takes about two weeks and is expensive.*

32. **Incompetent Cervix:** *An incompetent cervix, also called cervical insufficiency, is a condition that occurs when weak cervical tissue causes or contributes to premature birth or the loss of an otherwise healthy pregnancy.*

33. **Infertility:** *A disease of the reproductive system defined by the failure to achieve a clinical pregnancy after 12 months or more of regular unprotected sexual intercourse for women <35 years, and 6 months for women > 35 years.*

34. **Intubate:** *To put a tube in, commonly used to refer to the insertion of a breathing tube into the trachea for mechanical ventilation. For example, as a life-saving measure, an emergency room physician might intubate a patient who is not breathing adequately so that the lungs can be ventilated.*

35. **Intrauterine Insemination (IUI) / Artificial Insemination:** *A type of artificial insemination—is a procedure for treating infertility. Sperm that have been washed and concentrated are placed directly in your uterus around the time your ovary releases one or more eggs to be fertilized. Older types of artificial insemination placed the sperm in the vagina. While this was easier, it was not as successful as the current procedure.*

36. **Intravenous (IV):** *1) Into a vein. Intravenous (IV) medications are a solutions administered directly into the venous circulation via a syringe or intravenous catheter (tube). 2) The actual solution that is administered intravenously. 3) The device used to administer an intravenous solution, such as the familiar IV drip.*

37. **IV Push:** *A one time, rapid injection of medication into the bloodstream.*

38. **Laparoscopy / Laparoscopic Procedure:** *A laparoscopy/laparoscopic procedure is a type of surgery in which small incisions are made in the abdominal wall through which a laparoscope and other instruments can be placed to permit structures within the abdomen and pelvis to be seen. A variety of*

probes or other instruments can also be pushed through these small incisions in the skin. In this way, a number of surgical procedures can be performed without the need for a large surgical incision. Visualization is attained by the infusion of Carbon dioxide gas into the abdomen.

39. **Leiomyosarcoma:** *Often known as sarcoma, Leiomyosarcoma, is a very rare and aggressive cancer that can be found inside fibroid tumors, derived from smooth muscle cells typically of uterine, gastrointestinal or soft tissue origin. Leiomyosarcomas spread quickly and carry a poor prognosis.*

40. **Lupron:** *Lupron (leuprolide) overstimulates the body's own production of certain hormones, which causes that production to shut down temporarily. It is a medication often used to shrink fibroids and can cause menopausal symptoms.*

41. **Lysteda:** *Lysteda (tranexamic acid) is a man-made form of an amino acid (protein) called lysine. Tranexamic acid prevents enzymes in the body from breaking down blood clots. Lysteda is used to treat heavy menstrual bleeding.*

42. **Magnesium Sulfate:** *Magnesium is a mineral involved in many processes in the body including nerve signaling, the*

building of healthy bones, and normal muscle contraction. About 350 enzymes are known to depend on magnesium.

43. **Magnetic Resonance Imaging (MRI):** *Magnetic resonance imaging (MRI) is a technique that uses a magnetic field and radio waves to create detailed images of the organs and tissues within your body. Most MRI machines are large, tube-shaped magnets. When you lie inside an MRI machine, the magnetic field temporarily realigns hydrogen atoms in your body. Radio waves cause these aligned atoms to produce very faint signals, which are used to create cross-sectional MRI images—like slices in a loaf of bread.*

44. **Meconium:** *A dark, sticky material that is normally present in the intestine at birth and passed in the feces after birth. The passage of meconium before birth can be a sign of fetal distress.*

45. **Midwife:** *A trained person who assists women during childbirth. Many midwives also provide <u>prenatal care</u> for pregnant women, birth education for women and their partners, and care for mothers and newborn babies after the birth. Depending on local law, midwives may deliver babies in the*

*mother's home, in a birthing center or clinic, or in a hospital.
Most midwives specialize in normal, uncomplicated deliveries, referring women with health problems that could require
hospitalization during birth to a hospital-based obstetrician.
Others work with physicians as part of a team. Legal qualifications required to practice midwifery differ among the US
states and various countries.*

46. **Miscarriage:** *Loss of an embryo or fetus before the 20th
week of pregnancy. Most miscarriages occur during the first
14 weeks of pregnancy. The medical term for miscarriage is
spontaneous abortion.*

47. **Myomectomy:** *Myomectomy is an open surgical procedure
to remove uterine fibroids—also called leiomyomas.*

48. **MyoSure Tissue Removal System:** *A hysteroscopic procedure that can eliminate submucosal fibroids in the uterine
cavity without having to cut or remove any part of the uterus.*

49. **Nasogastric Tube (NG):** *A tube that is passed through the
nose and down through the nasopharynx and esophagus into
the stomach. Abbreviated NG tube. It is a flexible tube made
of rubber or plastic and can be used to remove the contents of*

the stomach, including air, to decompress the stomach, or to remove small solid objects and fluid, such as poison, from the stomach. An NG tube can also be used to put substances into the stomach, and so it may be used to place nutrients directly into the stomach when a patient cannot take food or drink by mouth.

50. **Neonatal Intensive Care Unit (NICU):** *An intensive care unit designed for premature and ill newborn babies.*

51. **Nitrazine Paper:** *A test paper made to turn from yellowish green to dark blue when it comes in contact with amniotic fluid.*

52. **NPO—Nothing by mouth:** *A medically approved abbreviation that means NOTHING BY MOUTH. The abbreviation is based on the Latin translation of "nil per os" meaning nothing by mouth. Often ordered prior to undergoing surgery.*

53. **NSAID:** *Nonsteroidal anti-inflammatory drug, a medication that is commonly prescribed or purchased over the counter to treat the inflammation associated with conditions such as arthritis, tendonitis, and bursitis. Examples of NSAIDs*

include aspirin, ibuprofen, and naproxen. Side effects including gastro intestinal bleeding, especially when taken on an empty stomach.

54. **Obstetrician:** *A physician who has successfully completed specialized education and training in the management of pregnancy, labor, and pueperium (the time-period directly following childbirth). An obstetrician/gynecologist is a physician specialist who provides medical and surgical care to women and has particular expertise in pregnancy, childbirth, and disorders of the reproductive system. This includes preventative care, prenatal care, detection of sexually transmitted diseases, Pap test screening, family planning, etc.*

55. **Obstetrics and Gynecology (OB/GYN):** *OB is short for obstetrics or for an obstetrician, a physician who delivers babies. GYN is short for gynecology or for a gynecologist, a physician who specializes in treating diseases of the female reproductive organs. The word "gynecology" comes from the Greek gyno, gynaikos meaning woman + logia meaning study, so gynecology literally is the study of women. These days gynecology is focused largely on disorders of the female reproductive organs. An obstetrician/gynecologist (OB/GYN) is therefore a physician who both delivers babies and treats diseases of the female reproductive organs.*

56. **Oncology:** *The field of medicine that is devoted to cancer. Clinical oncology consists of three primary disciplines: medical oncology (the treatment of cancer with medicine, including chemotherapy), surgical oncology (the surgical aspects of cancer including biopsy, staging, and surgical resection of tumors), and radiation oncology (the treatment of cancer with therapeutic radiation).*

57. **Operating Room (OR):** *A facility that is equipped for performing surgery.*

58. **Ovulation:** *The release of the ripe egg (ovum) from the ovary. The egg is released when the cavity surrounding it (the follicle) breaks open in response to a hormonal signal. Ovulation occurs around 14 or 15 days from the first day of the woman's last menstrual cycle. When ovulation occurs, the ovum moves into the Fallopian tube and becomes available for fertilization.*

59. **Oximetery:** *A procedure for measuring the concentration of oxygen in the blood. The test is used in the evaluation of various medical conditions that affect the function of the heart and lungs. The oximeters most commonly used today are called pulse oximeters because they respond only to pulsations, such as those in pulsating capillaries of the area tested.*

60. **Placenta Previa:** *Placenta previa occurs when a baby's placenta partially or totally covers the opening in the mother's cervix—the lower end of the uterus that connects to the top of the vagina. Placenta previa can cause severe bleeding before or during delivery.* This condition precludes a patient from having a vaginal delivery.

61. **Polycystic Ovarian Syndrome (PCOS):** *A common endocrine system disorder among women of reproductive age. Women with PCOS may have enlarged ovaries that contain small collections of fluid—called follicles—located in each ovary as seen during an ultrasound exam. Women with PCOS often have a more difficult time achieving pregnancy.*

62. **Post-Op/Post Operation:** *Pertaining to the period of time after surgery. It begins with the patient's emergence from anesthesia and continues through the time required for the acute effects of the anesthetic and surgical procedures to abate.*

63. **Pre-Term Delivery / Premature Birth:** *A pre-term delivery is defined as a delivery performed before 37 weeks of pregnancy are completed. I think this one line is enough. The sub-categories of a pre-term delivery, based on gestational age are: extremely preterm (<28 weeks), very preterm (28 to <32 weeks) and, moderate to late preterm (32 to <37 weeks).*

Induction or caesarean birth should not be planned before 39 completed weeks unless medically indicated.

64. **Preeclampsia:** *A pregnancy complication characterized by high blood pressure and signs of damage to another organ system, often the kidneys. Preeclampsia usually begins after 20 weeks of pregnancy in a woman whose blood pressure had been normal. Even a slight rise in blood pressure may be a sign of preeclampsia. Treatment for this condition is delivery of the fetus.*

65. **Premature Rupture of Membranes (PROM):** *A condition where fluid leaks from your amniotic sac before labor begins. The amniotic sac contains fluid that surrounds and protects your unborn baby in your uterus. If PROM happens before 37 weeks of pregnancy, it is called preterm PROM.*

66. **Prognosis:** *The forecast of the probable outcome or course of a disease; the patient's chance of recovery.*

67. **Prolapse:** *A condition where organs, such as the uterus, fall down or slip out of place. It is used for organs protruding through the vagina or the rectum or for the misalignment of the valves of the heart.*

68. **Radiographic Contrast Dye / Radiocontrast Agent:** *A type of medical contrast medium used to improve the visibility of internal bodily structures in X-ray-based imaging techniques such as computed tomography (CT), radiography, and fluoroscopy. Radiocontrast agents are typically iodine or barium compounds.*

69. **Reversal of End Diastolic Flow:** *Reversal of end diastolic flow (REDF) or velocity in umbilical arterial flow assessment is often an ominous finding if detected after 16 weeks. It signifies improper and insufficient flow to the baby and delivery is often warranted.*

70. **Robotic Myomectomy:** *A minimally invasive way for surgeons to remove uterine fibroids. The robotic platform allows for 3-dimensional visualization and enhanced wrist movement to perform delicate surgery.*

71. **Small Intestine Obstruction:** *Intestinal obstruction is a blockage that keeps food or liquid from passing through your small intestine or large intestine (colon). Intestinal obstruction may be caused by fibrous bands of tissue in the abdomen (adhesions), which form after surgery, inflamed or infected pouches in your intestine (diverticulitis), hernias and tumors. Without treatment, the blocked parts of the intestine can lose*

bloody supply and die. However, with prompt medical care, intestinal obstruction often can be successfully treated.

72. **Sonogram:** *An image produced by ultrasonography. Also called echogram, sonograph, ultrasonogram.*

73. **Spinal Meningitis:** *Inflammation of the membranes enclosing the spinal cord. If not treated quickly, it can be fatal.*

74. **Uterine Artery Embolization (UAE):** *Uterine Artery Embolization (UAE) is a minimally invasive treatment for uterine fibroids, noncancerous growths in the uterus. In uterine artery embolization—also called uterine fibroid embolization (UFE)—a doctor uses a slender, flexible tube (catheter) to inject small particles (embolic agents) into the uterine arteries, which supply blood to your fibroids and uterus. It is often used in peri-menopausal women who want to avoid hysterectomy.*

75. **Ultrasound:** *Diagnostic ultrasound, also called sonography or diagnostic medical sonography, is an imaging method that uses high-frequency sound waves to produce images of structures within your body. The images can provide valuable in-*

formation for diagnosing and treating a variety of diseases and conditions.

76. **Uterus / Uterine Lining:** *A hollow, pear-shaped organ that is located in a woman's lower abdomen, between the bladder and the rectum. It is a muscular organ that carries a growing baby. The narrow lower portion of the uterus is the cervix (the neck of the uterus). The broader upper part is the corpus, which is made up of three layers of tissue. In women of child-bearing age, the inner layer (endometrium) of the uterus goes through a series of monthly changes known as the menstrual cycle. Each month, endometrial tissue grows and thickens in preparation to receive a fertilized egg. Menstruation occurs when this tissue is not used, disintegrates, and passes out through the vagina. The middle layer (myometrium) of the uterus is muscular tissue that expands during pregnancy to hold the growing fetus and contracts during labor to deliver the child. The outer layer (parametrium) also expands during pregnancy and contracts thereafter.*

77. **Viable / Pre-viable:** *Viable is defined as being physically fitted to live, or (of a fetus) having reached such a stage of development as to be capable of living, under normal conditions, outside the uterus. Viability is defined between 23-24*

weeks of gestation. Pre-viable before the time at which the fetus is capable of maintaining a separate existence.

78. **Vitals:** *Those bodily organs that are essential to life, as the brain, heart, liver, lungs, and stomach.*

ABOUT THE AUTHORS

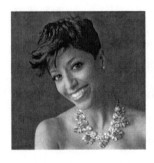 **Gessie J. Thompson**—New York-based Brand Strategist, Fibroids Advocate and Fertility Coach Gessie Thompson helps women and men navigate the challenges they encounter to conceive or carry their dreams to full term. As a Fertility Coach, she supports them to overcome the emotional and mental hurdles that accompany fibroids and infertility. As a Brand Strategist, she partners with entrepreneurs to package and give "birth" to their visions so they are positioned to change the world with their unique voice and message.

A founding board member of The White Dress Project—a non-profit dedicated to raising funds for research and awareness for uterine fibroids—Gessie has been a featured speaker on Fibroids and Fertility at ESSENCE Festival. Her story has been profiled in *ESSENCE* and she has appeared on "The Yolanda Adams Morning Show," "The Tom Joyner Morning Show," ARISE TV, *Hope for Women*, "The Frank Ski Morning Show" and more. Follow her at @gessieTUG and learn more about her at GessieThompson.com.

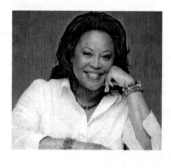

Coach Felicia T. Scott—Coach Felicia was selected from over a 1,000 speakers, to become eWomenNetwork's first "North America's Next Greatest Speaker." Touted as one of "today's leading motivational speakers," the Certified Empowerment Coach™ and bestselling author of *THRIVE!* designs, executes and administers emotional intelligence-based coaching and training programs that teach people how to optimize their performance.

In her ten-plus years working with Fortune 500 companies, executives, business leaders and entrepreneurs the ESSENCE.com Empowerment Columnist has helped thousands through her speaking, coaching, workshops and writing to unlock their strengths, live fearlessly, expand their leadership and, enjoy authentic and effective communication. She has appeared on ABC, FOX, BET, ARISE and more. Learn more about her at coachfelicia.com and follow her @AskCoachFelicia.

Join the "Circle of Hope" Prayer Group

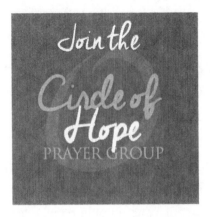

My Dear Hope Sister,

I believe hopelessness is the single-most deadly threat facing you in your battle for your miracle baby. This is why I started the "Circle of Hope" Prayer Call to encourage and inspire women like you to press on in pursuing your dream of motherhood. If you're struggling with fibroids, infertility or any other complications, join us for our next prayer call.

I know that, even when loved ones and family surround you, you sometimes feel alone because it seems no one understands what you're going through. But you're not! You have a network of sisters traveling your same journey who are waiting to support you with their prayers, testimonies, resources, victories and even tears.

When I felt like giving up, the prayers of my community encouraged me and together we warred for my baby! With their support, I learned that if I could just stay HOPE-FILLED, I could fight another day!

We connect for one hour every first and third Saturday of the month at 8 AM EST and we're here to stand in the gap for and with you for your miracle baby! Sign up to receive the call in details at gessiethompson.com/HopePrayer.

Your HOPE sister,

GessieThompson.com | @GessieTUG

Helps Us Secure A Presidential Proclamation Declaring July Fibroids Awareness Month!

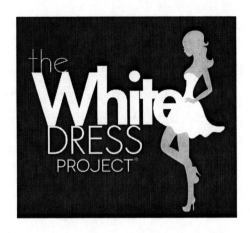

After ESSENCE published "My Fertility Journey" in the May 2014 issue, the accolades were overwhelming—over 33,000 women responded to it on Facebook and over 600 women thanked me for sharing my story because it gave them HOPE that they too could overcome fibroids. It was then that I realized how much women suffer from fibroids silently and became impassioned to become a Fibroids Awareness Advocate.

To that end, I became a spokesperson and board member of The White Dress Project (TWDP)—a non-profit committed to raising awareness and funds for research to fight the fibroids epidemic that plagues an astronomical 80% of black women, 70% of white women and 60% of Hispanic and Asian women by age 50.

Together with TWDP, we have helped make great strides in the battle against fibroids. In 2014, July was declared "Fibroids Awareness Month" in Georgia. In 2015, Florida and Louisiana were added to that list and resolutions are pending in the District of Columbia and Maryland. The Georgia House of Representatives Resolution 612 for a "Study Committee on Fibroids Awareness and Education" was passed and adopted in the same year. And, Congressman David Scott (GA-13) introduced a Congressional House resolution proclaiming July Fibroids Awareness Month nationally in the U.S. House of Representatives. Our next major milestone is to secure a presidential proclamation recognizing July as Fibroids Awareness Month and we need your help! Visit TheWhiteDressProject.com to sign the petition and learn more about how you can support the fight to prevent fibroids!

WhiteDressProject.com | @WeCanWearWhite

My Gift to You...

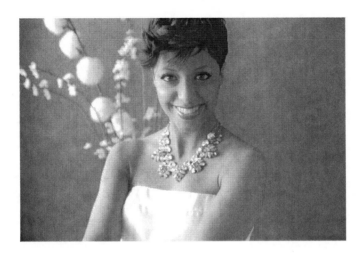

As my thanks for allowing me to be a part of your journey, I've recorded a special message just for you. It's called HOPE for the Journey Meditations! In it, I share what I believe are the three most important things you need to know as you press on in your fight for your miracle baby!

Download Your FREE
HOPE for the Journey Meditations MP3 at
GessieThompson.com/HopeMP3

CPSIA information can be obtained at www.ICGtesting.com
Printed in the USA
LVOW10s1610120216

474868LV00017B/1174/P

FEB 2 ⌂ 2016